# Praise for Nina Planck and *Real Food: What to Eat and Why*

"Persuasive and invigorating."

—**Michael Pollan**

"Compellingly smart."

—**Mark Bittman**

"The antidote to the faddists, alarmists, and kooks who all too often dominate American food discourse."

—**David Kamp, author of *The United States of Arugula***

"A cross between Alice Waters and Martha Stewart."

—**Jonathan Yardley, *The Washington Post***

"Who understands real food better than farmers themselves? Growing up on her parents' Virginia farm, Nina has lived the healthy benefits. How lucky then—ten years later—that *Real Food* continues to gain momentum."

—**Forrest Pritchard, organic farmer and *New York Times* bestselling author of *Gaining Ground***

"Nina Planck knows from real food."

—**CleanPlates.com**

"[*Real Food*] poses a convincing alternative to the prevailing dietary guidelines, even those treated as gospel . . . [Planck's] capacity for humor and self-deprecation makes for good company, and her intelligence and skepticism inspire confidence."

—**Holly Brubach, *The New York Times***

"The Frances Moore Lappé of her generation."

—***The Milkweed***

"Eating is our most fundamental and sensual act. It never did make sense to me that eating what's good for you should mean depriving yourself of foods you desire. Now Nina Planck explains

exactly why we are drawn to foods that delight our senses and keep us healthy."

—**Bill Niman, founder of Niman Ranch**

"Nina looks good in her overalls and tiara. As foodie royalty, she dispenses the practical and pragmatic with equal grace. I am a happier and healthier fellow thanks to her."

—**Paco Underhill, author of *Why We Buy: The Science of Shopping***

"Long before #hashtags were a thing, Nina was educating us on the value of #realfood. She was way ahead of the curve."

—**Marco Canora, author of *A Good Food Day* and *Brodo: A Bone Broth Cookbook***

"Nina Planck's journey—from rebellious farm girl to suave intellectual vegetarian to protective meat-eating mom—affirms everything that is sacred and right about food. If I were in a quandary about what kind of food to buy, I would read *Real Food* and quit wondering."

—**Joel Salatin, author of *Folks, This Ain't Normal***

"We met Nina a little over ten years ago, when she was heading up the Greenmarket Farmers Markets in New York City . . . Her knowledge about the many facets of food is vast and we have learned so much from her in the intervening years."

—**HandpickedNation.com**

REAL FOOD FOR MOTHER AND BABY

# REAL FOOD
## for MOTHER and BABY

*The Fertility Diet, Eating for Two,*
*and Baby's First Foods*

## NINA PLANCK

BLOOMSBURY
NEW YORK · LONDON · OXFORD · NEW DELHI · SYDNEY

Bloomsbury USA
An imprint of Bloomsbury Publishing Plc

| | |
|---|---|
| 1385 Broadway | 50 Bedford Square |
| New York | London |
| NY 10018 | WC1B 3DP |
| USA | UK |

www.bloomsbury.com

BLOOMSBURY and the Diana logo are trademarks of Bloomsbury Publishing Plc

First published 2009
This paperback edition published 2016

ISBN: PB: 978-1-63286-459-8
ebook: 978-1-63286-571-7

LIBRARY OF CONGRESS CATALOGING-IN-PUBLICATION DATA
Planck, Nina, 1971–
Real food for mother and baby : the fertility diet, eating for two, and
baby's first foods / Nina Planck.
p. cm.
Includes bibliographical references.
ISBN: 978-1-63286-459-8 (PB) 978-1-63286-571-7 (ebook)
1. Pregnancy—Nutritional aspects—Popular works. 2. Fertility,
Human—Nutritional aspects—Popular works. 3. Infants—Nutrition—
Popular works. I. Title.
RG559.P53 2009
618.2'42—dc22
2008038866

2 4 6 8 10 9 7 5 3 1

Designed by Sara Stemen
Typeset by RefineCatch Limited, Bungay, Suffolk
Printed and bound in the U.S.A. by Berryville Graphics, Inc., Berryville, Virginia

To find out more about our authors and books visit www.bloomsbury.com. Here you will find extracts, author interviews, details of forthcoming events, and the option to sign up for our newsletters.

Bloomsbury books may be purchased for business or promotional use. For information on bulk purchases please contact Macmillan Corporate and Premium Sales Department at specialmarkets@macmillan.com.

Were they called upon to name the most important factor in contributing to the healthy development of the human conceptus, most authorities would unhesitatingly declare for the good nutrition status of the mother.

—Ashley Montagu, *Prenatal Influences*, 1962

# Contents

# Foreword

I picked up *Real Food for Mother and Baby* when my son Lorenzo, my first, was eight months old. I come from an old-school Italian family. Everybody was telling me to put cereal in Lorenzo's bottle so that he would sleep better and gain more weight. Babies try to tell you what they need, and my understanding of what he was telling me was that he needed protein and fat: he loved my milk; he loved egg yolks, avocado, and rich meat. Nina confirmed what I thought and what I felt.

Now I'm the executive director of Choices in Childbirth, which works to demystify pregnancy and birth, and make sure women have access to safe, healthy, and respectful maternity care. We hear from many women who think and feel one way, yet are being told something different. Like Nina, we validate maternal instincts with clear information, so women can make good decisions for themselves and their babies.

I love that Nina devotes a full chapter to breastmilk, which is as real as real food gets. Too many mothers choose breast-feeding, but don't get the support they need. Hospital nurses still shame women by asking them to "cover up." New mothers are prevented from holding their babies for hours following a cesarean section, which works against easy breast-feeding. Mothers who must return to work tell us they couldn't afford a pump or were never taught how to use one. Furthermore, it's nigh impossible to go back to work six weeks after birth if you want to continue to breast-feed. We need more people like

Nina to make the case for feeding our babies the best food we have.

Pregnancy and new motherhood are sensitive times. People dispense a million pieces of advice: eat this, not that; graze, have a big dinner; eat fruit, or don't. Never mind the chatter. Nina tell us something else: relax, and be a normal human. Eat well, but enjoy yourself. Have a glass of wine, have a piece of chocolate, give your kid ketchup.

*Real Food for Mother and Baby* gives women a refreshing perspective on how to feed our bodies, ourselves, our babies, and our families. She also gives a bracing lesson on what *not* to worry about. Just get back to basics: meat, dairy, fish, greens, and whole grains. Never preachy, Nina liberates us to do the best we can, without anxiety or guilt.

Ultimately Nina teaches us how to combine quality food with the good life. All that real food, including real ice cream and dark chocolate, adds up over time, making our kids better off and our lives sweeter.

Michele Giordano
Choices in Childbirth
New York City
January 2016

# Introduction

It's a damp and chilly day in late November, and I'm marveling that I'm here in my little office on Prince Street, typing with two hands like any other person with a job—that is, without a little squirming guy on my lap. Our son Julian is more than a year old, a sturdy thing, and just now he's off having adventures with his lovely babysitter, Judy. Maybe he's transfixed by one of the many charming dogs on the streets of New York City, or spinning his plump finger to say he's spied a fan. Perhaps he's shouting at a big dirty garbage truck groaning down the street.

Julian still nurses every day, but I'm dressed like a normal person and feel like one, too. I'm wearing a nice bra, not some maternity number. My breasts are not swollen, leaking, or aching. I have a strange, happy sensation of being grown-up. I'm older and wiser, but not sadder. Somewhat to my surprise, I'm as healthy as ever in all the ways I can count: lean, fit, well rested, cheerful.

They say the first year rushes by in a blur. For me every episode is still vivid. I can picture my thirty-four-hour labor, hour by hour. I can still see the apartment, after I'd labored in every possible position and location, as if the place had been ransacked by burglars after cash. I remember the first thrilling night alone with Julian, and I remember other nights alone, less thrilling, when he nursed, lost his milk, nursed, and lost his milk—again and again. "Who will feed *me*?" I asked the room.

Julian may not remember his first snowstorm, first trip to a Christmas tree farm, first pee in the potty, or first encounter with the steaming nostril of a horse, but I do. When Julian was eight months old, he donned a gray windbreaker and boarded a four-seater plane. The unflappable baby took a good look at the sea as we gained altitude and then nursed calmly. When the tiny plane landed gently on a grass runway in the woods on Waldron, we climbed out unruffled and boarded a 1953 flatbed Ford, for a tour of organic farms in the San Juan Islands. Julian used his potty next to a vegetable patch.

That summer, Rob and I schlepped all over Manhattan, from the Upper West Side to TriBeCa, test-driving pediatricians. At his nine-month visit, Julian kept "failing." Three doctors in two days asked the same questions. Does he wave bye-bye? No. Clap hands? No. Say "mama" and "dada"? No. We hung our heads. It's tough to have a backward son in a city of future Nobel winners, still wearing short pants. But even the Pediatrician Tour was comic, not nerve-wracking. Julian didn't clap, but he could catch a beetle lickety-split. Our first year with Julian was full of easy adventures.

There is a culture of worry, hardship, and complaint around pregnancy, birth, and motherhood. It's a culture I want no part of. It's boring. It's self-absorbed. It's whiny. Worse, it mars what's rightly a celebration. However, I do appreciate that this same culture reflects reality. Some pregnant and nursing women don't feel so great. That's a shame. I think they could feel better.

I loved being pregnant with Julian. I was on a book tour in months six, seven, and eight. I was still jogging at thirty-nine weeks and back to running again not long after the birth. Three weeks after Julian was born, he went with me to give a talk about real food. He quietly nursed while I signed books. When he was two months old, we took two trains to Virginia without a hitch. When I turned thirty-six, Julian was five months old and I was in my prepregnancy jeans. At one year, I feel great.

Good luck? Good genes? No doubt a bit of both. But I do have one tip. I ate real food, lots of it. The benefits of real food start with conception. It's easier to get pregnant if you're eat-ing right. Some of the minor complaints of pregnancy, such as swelling, can be avoided by eating well. Real food can ease the early challenges of motherhood, such as the baby blues. Later, many mothers waste precious time following pointless advice about baby's first foods.

The popular pregnancy books I read didn't seem to know these things. They didn't understand real food, and they had other advice for pregnant women I thought was balderdash. So I did my own homework on foods for fertility, pregnancy, and weaning. What I learned is in your hands. So is eating well.

It's nice to be in control of lunch, because most of mother-hood you cannot plan for. Mothers did warn me. When I got preg-nant, my friend Terry said, "There will be a new Nina. And the old Nina will never come back." This seemed rather bleak. At the time, I was somewhat attached to the person she was blithely calling "the old Nina." In *The Big Book of Birth*, Erica Lyon is equally direct. "When we give birth for the first time, *there is a death*. Immediate and sudden."

Now I understand. Motherhood changes you. Your body is never the same. Your time is not your own. Everyone has her pleasures. Maybe yours is a deep bath, a long weekend run, knead-ing bread, or three hours in bed with a novel. After the baby, these dispensable activities get short shrift, certainly at first, maybe for a while.

Don't despair. Your body will be different, probably forever, but that doesn't necessarily mean it's worse. As for the time spent reveling in what looks like unfettered independence, pleasing myself at will and repeatedly, I had my years. I don't miss it.

That said, your new body, the way you spend the day—dramatic as they seem—are merely superficial modifications. Ev-eryone knows a new baby is coming. Even you, in your most befuddled, I-can't-believe-I'm-pregnant moments, know that. It's more difficult to grasp that another version of *you* is coming, too. Not one fixed version. The new you is flickering, mutable. When I was pregnant, I often thought, *So this is me, pregnant. I like me, pregnant.* Three weeks later, things were different: my body, feelings, outlook. Each time I got used to myself, I vanished from view.

When your baby is born, of course, there is a great lurch in identity. One day, you're "just" pregnant, almost like any other citizen without kids. The next day, you're a Mother. Now dawns a new string of changes, often subtle, in body and mind. Who is she, this new you? No one knows. Not the baby's father. Not your best friend, doctor, minister, rabbi, or shrink. You'll probably be the last to find out.

The best preparation for pregnancy, birth, and mothering— even better than real food—is an open mind. Perhaps your life and work are well planned, orderly. Perhaps you find that satisfying. (I did.) Let go. Having a baby is stupendously wonderful, but things may not go as planned. If you have no fixed expectations, nothing can surprise or disappoint you. The ideal stance is a kind of gentle wonder, now and again brimming over into radical amazement, as your story unfolds.

New York City
November 2008

## CHAPTER 1

# What Is Real Food?

### REAL FOOD DEFINED

Before we look at what to eat and why, let me define real food. Later, when I say, "eat fish," you'll know what kind of fish to eat. Mothers, fathers, and babies will all benefit from eating real food. So will grandfathers and grandmothers, aunts, uncles, teenagers, and children, come to think of it. This primer works for anyone who eats.

My definition of real food is based on science, but it's not meant to be technical. It's meant to be memorable. It's short-hand, a rule of thumb, a principle to live by. If you can master this two-part description of real food, this could be the last book on nutrition you ever pick up. Here goes: *Real food is old and it's traditional.*

"Old" means we've been eating these foods for a long time. Let's take a vastly simplified view of our diet and divide it roughly into two periods: the Paleolithic (Stone Age) and the Neolithic (the farming era). Anything you can hunt, fish, or gather is a Stone Age food. Meat, fish, fowl, insects, eggs, leaves, nuts, berries, and even the odd sip of honey made up meals for our hunter-gatherer ancestors. We've been eating beef and venison for a very long time—at least one or two million years—while fish and fowl are somewhat more recent. Cultivated foods, such as wheat, rice, beans, and things we make from them, such as bread, wine, and beer, are considerably more recent. We started to eat these foods about ten thousand years ago, when, gradually, we began to tend crops.

Dairy foods fall somewhere in the middle. Many people think that milk is a farming-era food, but that's probably mistaken. Humans were probably herding, and even breeding, grazing mammals to secure a more reliable supply of fresh milk before they settled down to farm properly. The misconception that milk comes with farming probably has to do with the modern industrial practice—a bad one—of feeding grain to cattle. The natural diet of cattle is grass, not corn and soybeans. Because grass was abundant before we got handy growing, threshing, and storing grain, it's more likely that shepherds were grazing goats, sheep, and cows on grass before crop farming was common. From the clues we have, it could be that herding, and thus fresh milk consumption, is about thirty thousand years old. Cheese, yogurt, and butter are also old foods. We've used fresh milk in the same basic recipes for at least five thousand years.

The Old Foods Pantry is ample and diverse. Meat, fish, poultry, milk, cheese, yogurt, nuts, berries, potatoes, leaves, lentils, chick peas, honey—and their close relations—are all old foods of good standing in our diet. If you're wondering what food *wouldn't* qualify, consider these more recent foods, along with a rough estimate of their regular appearance in the human diet: white sugar (1600s), margarine made from vegetable oil (1900s), and corn syrup (1970s).

Real food is also traditional. By that I mean it's produced and prepared roughly as it once was, before factories gave us lesser versions. Real milk and eggs are whole and fresh, real beef is grass fed, and real orange juice is raw. It was ever thus. Industrial food cuts corners, giving us spray-dried skim milk powder and pasteurized egg whites, grain-fed beef, and pasteurized orange juice. Nutrition and flavor are lost.

Imitation is the hallmark of industrial food. Instead of traditional milk, the food industry will sell you soybean juice tarted up with brown rice syrup and vanilla. Instead of cheese made with whole milk, salt, and cultures, they'll sell you vegetable oil and water mixed with orange dye and additives to give it a cheese-like look and feel. Instead of butter, they'll sell you corn oil pummeled with hydrogen atoms to make it solid at room temperature, dye it yellow, and call it "buttery."

Traditional foods are whole, complete, intact. A pork chop with the fat, brown rice, and an orange are whole. Industrial foods are broken, incomplete. That includes whey powder, isolated soybean protein, and "baby" carrot cores, foods our ancestors never saw. They had whole milk, tofu, and grown-up carrots. Food the food industry has fiddled with isn't whole. That's why I don't buy things that are engineered to be low in one thing or high in another: no high-protein bars, low-carbohydrate bread, low-fat cheese. I don't eat foods that have been broken down into their component parts and reassembled, such as skim milk powder reconstituted with water. I don't buy foods missing good stuff we want. If meat is naturally lean, like wild venison, that's fine, but I ignore the advice to "choose lean meat." In our house, we trim the steak to taste.

Stripped-down foods are inferior. The food industry knows this. That's why it adds back the B vitamins missing from white flour. That's why the law requires synthetic vitamin D, which is naturally found in butterfat, in skim milk. Apple peels contain up to 40 percent of the antioxidant flavonoids in an apple and about one third of the vitamin C.[1] Broccoli and pomegranate—not extracts of broccoli and pomegranate—fight cancer; eating whole grains, not cereal fiber, reduces mortality in women.[2]

Just as you would eat the whole apple, I recommend you eat the whole beast. I call this "whole meat." If you eat skinless, boneless chicken breast, you get the muscle, which is good, but you miss the nutrients in the skin, bone, and fat. Certain amino acids (methionine) are found in muscle, while others are found in the skin and bones (glycine). The fat in chicken skin and dark meat contains the antimicrobial fat palmitoleic acid. The bones contain calcium, the joints gelatin. There is more iron in marrow bone than in muscle.[3]

Traditional foods are diverse—as diverse as the climates where you find them, from the tropics to the Arctic Circle. Industrial food, by contrast, is monochromatic and getting more so. According to Michael Pollan, the best American chronicler of industrial foodways, just four crops—corn, rice, soy, wheat—account for two thirds of the calories we eat. If you eat industrial food, your diet is effectively reduced to the products that can be manufactured from these four plants. If you eat real food, your diet is virtually unlimited.

Traditional food is fundamentally conservative—it doesn't change—while industrial food changes relentlessly. The food industry gives us thousands of new foodlike products each year, each boasting its novelty, the better to boost profits. But many recipes made with real food haven't changed in thousands of years. We still make real yogurt the same way as always. You add cultures, famously *L. bulgaricus*, *S. thermophilus*, and *L. acidophilus*, to fresh milk. That's it. Adding flavor to yogurt is just as simple. Honey, nuts, and berries are the real foods I happen to like with yogurt.

Compare this with industrial yogurt. "Yogurt" made with soybeans speaks for itself. It must be industrial because it's an imitation, a fake. The latest "enhanced" yogurt contains omega-3 fats derived from algae. It cannot be traditional because it's engineered to be something it's not. The algae oil, which is patented by a biochemical company, has nothing to do with yogurt. Real yogurt does contain some omega-3 fats, if the cows were grass fed.

If you're muddled about whether the food you're pondering in aisle 6 is real or not, try this test. Does it look like the food your great-grandparents ate? It doesn't matter whether they came from England, Germany, and Sweden (like mine) or from Mexico,

Vietnam, Poland, Turkey, Nigeria, Boston, Talladega, or anywhere else. The menus from these places may vary, but before industrial food, the basic ingredients were remarkably similar.

The world over, cooks used grass-fed and pastured meat, poultry, and eggs; wild fish, lightly cooked and often raw; full-fat dairy from grass-fed cows, sheep, or goats, including butter, whole milk, and raw milk cheese; whole grains and legumes, often soaked or fermented; ecological fruit and vegetables; pure maple syrup and raw honey; and traditional fats and oils, such as butter, lard, and coconut oil. These ingredients are old, traditional, and whole.

Recipes made from real food are also real foods. Sausage made with fresh pork, herbs, spices, and natural casing is real food. Mayonnaise made with egg yolks, olive oil, salt, and a dash of mustard is real food. Soaked lentils simmered with pancetta are real food. Fermented and cultured foods, such as yogurt, miso, and bread made with whole grains and yeast or sourdough, are real. Ice cream made with milk, cream, peaches, and a small amount of sugar—an industrial food I find impossible to give up entirely—is real food. Ice cream with raw honey or pure maple syrup is even better. Dark chocolate is real food. So are coffee, tea, wine, and beer—all traditional fermented drinks. You can season real food with real salt. That means unrefined sea salt, which contains about eighty essential minerals and trace elements, including magnesium, potassium, and iodine.

Some real foods, such as red meat and butter, have been blamed for modern diseases, especially heart disease. More precisely, experts said that too much fat, and saturated fat in particular, was killing us. On closer inspection, this theory, known as the lipid hypothesis, has some notable weaknesses. One problem is timing. We've been eating pork and butter for millennia, but heart disease is a modern problem. The first heart attack was diagnosed in 1912. Epidemiological evidence also contradicts the assertion that traditional foods cause chronic metabolic conditions. People who (still) eat traditional diets, diets rich in real food—saturated coconut oil, whole milk, and red meat—don't get fat. They don't get diabetes and heart disease, either—that is, not until they switch to industrial foods, like white flour and corn oil.

The "less fat is better" message was misguided. Would you consider the Harvard University School of Public Health a credible witness to this public health debacle? "It is now increasingly recognized that the low-fat campaign has been based on little scientific evidence and may have caused unintended health problems," wrote Frank Hu and other Harvard researchers in the *Journal of the American College of Nutrition*. Only two studies found a "significant positive association between saturated fat intake and risk of CHD [coronary heart disease]," they noted, while many more failed to find such a link. This observation was made in 2001.

Recent research vindicates saturated fats. Writing in the *Annals of Internal Medicine* in 2014, Dr. Rajiv Chowdhury reported no link between saturated fats and heart disease after reviewing nearly eighty studies. When the researchers examined specific fatty acids in the blood, they found that margaric acid (a saturated fat found in butter) and omega-3 fats found in fish were associated with less cardiovascular risk. Two types of fats were associated with more heart disease: human-made trans fats and omega-6 fats, typically from grain and seed oils.

I have good news. Real food, including beef, butter, and eggs, won't kill you. Certain dieters may wish to note that good whole wheat bread won't hurt you either. Indeed real food may well contribute to a long life—and a happy one, if pleasure matters to you. As the journalist Nina Teicholz and others have demonstrated, myths about real food—chiefly, that natural saturated fats and cholesterol cause heart disease—are collapsing under the weight of evidence.[4]

Consider cholesterol. When dietary cholesterol was accused of causing heart disease, egg yolks got a bad reputation. It was undeserved. "Surprisingly, there is little direct evidence linking higher egg consumption and increased risk of CHD," Hu wrote in the same article just cited. Hu would know. In 1999, his own team cleared eggs in the *Journal of the American Medical Association*. A study of 118,000 people "found no evidence of an overall significant association between egg consumption" and heart disease.[5] In fact, people who ate five or six eggs a week had a lower risk of heart disease than those who ate less than one egg per week.

Natural cholesterol is actually good for you. Cholesterol plays many crucial roles in the body, including building sex hormones and brain cells. When you eat carbohydrate, your body breaks it down into simple sugars. It spends some sugar for energy, sends some to the brain, and stores what you don't need. Then the liver converts stored sugar into cholesterol and triglycerides. In modest amounts, that's healthy. But eating refined carbohydrates raises VLDL, the very dense lipoprotein associated with heart disease. Moreover, when you don't eat fresh cholesterol, your body produces more.

Here's a sampling of recent research on the crumbling low-fat theory. High "total" cholesterol is not a reliable predictor of heart disease; it's not even a major risk factor in women. Eating natural saturated fat raises HDL, which is good, while corn oil lowers HDL, which is bad. Eating saturated coconut oil improves the HDL ratio. Even "high" LDL is not always dangerous, although mucking about with it may be. Statins, the class of drugs that stops your liver from making LDL, deplete your body of the antioxidant coenzyme $Q_{10}$ ($CoQ_{10}$), which the heart muscle depends on.[6] In Wales, men who drink the most milk have the least stroke and heart disease. In Finland, researchers studied men who ate butter and whole milk and others who ate margarine and skim milk. The real food eaters had better cholesterol levels.

So why are we sick? Not because we eat real food, but because we don't. The main nutritional cause of obesity, diabetes, and heart disease is industrial food. Synthetic trans fats, not

natural saturated fats, cause heart disease. Eating too many vegetable oils (corn, sunflower, safflower, and soybean oil) and refined carbohydrates leads to weight gain, obesity, diabetes, and
heart disease. Deficiencies also contribute to heart disease. Two
nutrients notably missing in a diet of industrial food are B vitamins and omega-3 fats.

Obesity, diabetes, and heart disease are called the "diseases
of civilization," but I think this moniker is misleading. The ancient
Greeks were civilized, but they didn't succumb to these chronic
conditions. Industrial foods, foods we have been eating only recently, are to blame. I call obesity, diabetes, and heart disease the
"diseases of industrialization."

My advice here will be brief. First, learn to recognize industrial foods. They are new to the human diet. They rely on imitation to get your attention and respect. They are refined,
incomplete, broken. Once you're alert to industrial food, don't
bring it home. Don't buy it when you eat out. Don't feed it to
people you love. Second, buy the best real food you can afford.
It tastes better. And it's good for you.

## REAL MILK

I grew up on a vegetable farm in Virginia. Tomatoes, squash,
and peppers were the cash crops, but we also kept a somewhat
grumpy Jersey cow named Mabel for what we called "home
use." Milking was a family chore. It was a chore I hated fiercely.
Mabel often stepped in the bucket, and at school, I thought I
smelled like a cow. I didn't much care for a glass of milk,
either, although I always liked peaches mashed in milk. Now,
of course, I am altogether nostalgic about Mabel, milking,
and milk itself. I grew up drinking real milk—fresh, grass fed,
hormone free, full fat, raw, and unhomogenized—and that
makes me a lucky girl. Today, especially when I'm pregnant or
nursing and need the extra food, I drink extra milk and thrive
on it.

Unfortunately, it's not easy to find real milk. In some states, selling raw milk in shops is illegal. In others, you can buy it at the farm or via private arrangements. When we're at Small Farm we can cross the river to Pennsylvania to buy raw milk, but we also drink a lot of the best local pasteurized milk we can find. It's everything but raw: grass fed, hormone free, unhomogenized. We find good milk in the dairy case at Rob's shop, Murray's Cheese, in local health food shops, and at our local farmers' markets. All told, finding proper milk is getting easier. Here's what you need to know.

*Real milk is from grass-fed cows.* The natural diet of cows is forage: grass, hay, and other roughage. Industrial cows are fed on corn and soy and never go outside. We gave Mabel a scoop of grain at milking, and many grass farmers do the same. That's OK; even an ancient wild cow would have eaten some seed heads. Grass-fed milk and cream contain more omega-3 fats and vitamin E than grain-fed dairy products.

*Real milk comes from cows that are not treated with hormones.* Some cows are given recombinant bovine growth hormone (rBGH) to boost milk production. This milk contains higher levels of IGF-1, an insulin-like hormone, which is identical in cows and humans. IGF-1 causes cells to proliferate, and it's linked to cancer. When you drink milk from a cow treated with rBGH, you get a dose of IGF-1. Because the U.S. Food and Drug Administration (FDA) regards rBGH as safe for humans, it does not permit the words "hormone free" on milk labels, but most dairy farmers who don't use synthetic hormones find a way to say so. Many farmers are giving up rBGH because it shortens milking life and consumers don't want it. It's banned in Europe and Canada.

*Real milk is raw.* Pasteurization, or heat treatment, is used to kill pathogens in milk. Unfortunately, it also destroys a host of nutrients, including folic acid and vitamins A, $B_6$, and C. Heat inactivates the enzymes required to absorb nutrients in milk: lipase (to digest fats); lactase (to digest lactose); and phosphatase (to absorb calcium). The presence of phosphatase explains why raw milk contains more available calcium than pasteurized milk.[7] Pasteurization alters milk proteins and damages omega-3 fats. Heat also damages immune-boosting factors such as B-lymphocytes, macrophages, neutrophils, lymphocytes, and antibodies.

There are three kinds of pasteurization. Smaller dairies use two fairly gentle methods to preserve the taste and texture of milk. The vat method heats milk to about 145 degrees Fahrenheit for thirty minutes. The High Temperature Short Time method heats the milk to 162 degrees Fahrenheit for fifteen seconds. The harsh method is called ultrahigh temperature (UHT). Milk is heated briefly to 284 degrees Fahrenheit, rendering it completely sterile. When packaged in aseptic containers, unopened UHT milk is stable at room temperature for up to six months. That's good for shippers and retailers. But major nutrients, including protein and lactose, are damaged.[8] That's why you can't make good yogurt or cheese from UHT milk. It also has a pronounced cooked flavor.

*Real milk is not homogenized.* That means the cream rises to the top. To homogenize milk, the dairy industry forces the fat particles through a tiny screen until they are very small and evenly distributed throughout the milk. Cream-top milk has superior texture and flavor, and you can pour the cream off for special uses.

Organic milk is produced without hormones or pesticides. It contains more beneficial fats (CLA and omega-3) and more antioxidants than industrial milk. The organic label does *not* mean cows were grass-fed. Most organic cows eat lots of grain. Organic cows must have "access" to pasture, but on many large dairies, cows spend little time outside. Organic does not mean raw. Most commercial organic brands use the UHT method.

*Real milk is whole milk.* We never drink skim milk. Vitamins A and D are found in the fat, and you need both vitamins to absorb calcium. "The fat in whole milk also is present in the correct amount to promote the most efficient absorption of calcium," write Gail Sforza Brewer and the obstetrician Tom Brewer in *What Every Pregnant Woman Should Know*. Saturated fat in particular stimulates bone mineral density and bone growth.[9]

Industrial skim milk has another undesirable quality. To restore its "creamy" mouth feel and cover up its bluish color, the dairy industry adds whey proteins, such as alpha-lactalbumin, to skim. The effect is to tip the hormone balance to more male hormones. According to Jorge Chavarro, Walter C. Willett, and Patrick J. Skerrett in *The Fertility Diet*, the excess androgens in skim milk cause acne and ovulatory infertility. Drinking whole milk improves chances of conception.

Some people avoid milk, thinking they cannot digest the milk carbohydrate lactose. Although it's commonly called "lactose intolerance," this condition is more accurately described as insufficient lactase production. Lactase is the enzyme that breaks down lactose. Breast milk contains lactose, so babies make plenty of lactase to digest it. Lactase production tends to fall around the age of three or four, when babies were traditionally weaned.

If you continue to drink fresh milk past weaning, however, your body continues to make lactase. In many cultures, from Europe to Africa, including the Masai herding people of Kenya, adults drink milk. The ability to drink cow, sheep, and goat milk in adulthood—in other words, to produce lactase after age four—is so useful, this genetic mutation has evolved independently on several occasions in the last three thousand to seven thousand years.

Long ago, I thought I was lactose intolerant, but it was simply poor digestion, with multiple causes. Eating real food solved all my digestive trouble, and now I thrive on milk. If you have difficulty digesting fresh milk, consider cultured milks, such as cheese and yogurt. The lactose has already been digested by friendly bacteria. Raw milk, which contains the enzyme lactase, is preferable to pasteurized. I've known people who were flattened with stomach pain after drinking industrial milk who drank raw milk with ease.

Everything I've said about real milk is true of other dairy foods. Superior cheese, yogurt, butter, crème fraîche, sour cream, and other dairy products are made from real milk. I buy good versions of all of these foods, but with the exception of cheese, they are seldom made from raw milk. I don't worry about that. We buy plain whole milk yogurt with the cream on top and add our own honey or maple syrup. We buy all kinds of traditional cheeses, both raw milk and pasteurized.

Whey is another fine food and an easily digestible, liquid source of calcium and protein for pregnant women. You can buy whey from a farmer or make it at home, simply by straining whole milk yogurt through a clean cloth. In an hour or two, a quart of yogurt will yield about two cups of whey and a blob of dense, creamy yogurt.

Don't buy industrial dairy foods, such as powdered milk, which is made by spray-drying skim milk. This creates oxidized cholesterol, the only kind of cholesterol that's bad for you.

## A QUICK LOOK AT REAL MILK

| INDUSTRIAL MILK | ORGANIC MILK | REAL MILK |
|---|---|---|
| Corn, grain, and soybeans | Organic feed | Mostly grass and hay |
| Growth hormones | No hormones | No hormones |
| Cows indoors | Cows have "access" to pasture | Cows graze outside |
| Pasteurized | Pasteurized, often UHT | Raw or HTST-pasteurized |
| Homogenized | Sometimes homogenized | Unhomogenized |

Because it's cheap, powdered milk is often used in fluid skim milk. Unfortunately, the label doesn't disclose whether it's powdered milk or the real thing inside. On milk and many junk foods, the label will only say "skim milk." In my view, this scandal is reason enough never to drink skim. Don't buy powdered whey or protein drinks and bars made with it. To make whey protein, you start with whey or milk, filter it to remove the lactose, and then spray-dry it.

Naturally, I cannot recommend imitation dairy products, such as nondairy "creamer" or soybean juice. If you prefer not to drink milk for any reason, that's fine. Just don't! Many individuals, and indeed entire cultures, thrive without dairy products. It's quite possible to get all the nutrients you need from other foods, but not from soy.

## REAL MEAT, POULTRY, AND EGGS

My mother loves meat, always has. The Mother Goose rhyme about Hannah Bantry, alone in the pantry gnawing on a mutton bone, is perhaps her favorite. She'll often recite it mischievously as she picks up her own lamb chop. A few hours after I was born— in our old house in Buffalo, New York—my mother was ravenous for organic liver from Walnut Acres. With its Stone Age overtones, this meal became the stuff of family legend. Now I think of it as a self-administered iron transfusion to follow the immense exertion of giving birth. It was 1971, Walnut Acres was a pioneering organic brand, and my mother a real food pioneer.

Two years later, Dad gave up university life and my parents became farmers in Loudoun County, Virginia. For a good while money was tight, so I didn't grow up on organic meat, much less real meat, as I now define it. Now and then, local hunters brought us venison, but mostly we ate supermarket meat, including the less fancy cuts, like chicken liver. Only later, when times were better and there were more local farmers selling better stuff, did my parents buy superior grass-fed and pastured meats.

With a limited budget, you have to make choices, and I think my mother made the right ones. I would do the same in her shoes. Whole meat and poultry are some of the most nutritious foods you can eat, and the body needs protein every day. If price were an issue, I'd eat supermarket meat before junk deli meat, imitation meats made of soy protein, or no meat at all. Just buy the best meat you can afford.

Real meat starts with the natural diet of the animal. Cattle are herbivores. They can live on grass, leaves, stems, and nothing more. Thanks to the bacteria in their four stomachs, they can transform green things into meat and milk. That's true of all ruminants, including sheep, goats, and deer. A pig, on the other hand, is an omnivore. He'll eat anything, from milk to eggs, acorns to coconuts, but unlike a steer, he must have protein. Chickens and turkeys are omnivores, too. Knowing this much, you can decipher what's real food for each animal.

*Real beef and lamb are grass fed.* All animals start out on mother's milk and grass; the difference is whether they are fattened on grain or more grass. A little grain at the end is not so terrible, and it adds some very nice fat to a steak, but purists will insist on 100 percent grass-fed red meat. Industrial cattle are fattened in feedlots on grain and soybeans. If you can't find grass-fed beef, "vegetarian" beef is the next best thing. Cattle should not eat any animal products. Feeding parts of infected sheep and cattle to other cattle is what caused the mad cow disease crisis in Britain. Unfortunately, the U.S. beef industry hasn't absorbed the lessons of that disaster. That's why it's still legal to feed industrial poultry litter and restaurant plate waste to cattle here. Both may contain cattle parts, which makes carnivores of herbivores and breaks the fundamental rule of real meat: The animal eats its natural diet.

Grass-fed beef and lamb contain more omega-3 fats, vitamin E, beta-carotene, and CLA, an anticancer fat, than industrial meat. The beta-carotene makes real beef fat yellow, not white, like fat on a grain-fed steak. Grain-fed cattle are also more likely to carry a dangerous form of *E. coli*, called O157, than grass-fed cattle. That's because the grain diet makes their stomachs unnaturally acidic, an environment in which *E. coli* O157 thrives. There is normally a lot of (mostly benign) *E. coli* in the intestinal tract of a healthy steer, but O157 is more dangerous to humans because it can survive our acidic stomachs and make us sick.

*Real pork and poultry are pastured.* Look for pigs, chickens, and turkeys raised outdoors on pasture. They also eat corn and other foods, as nature intended, so we don't call them grass fed. "Free-range" means very little. Sometimes, a farmer says "free-range" when he means "pastured." But usually it merely means the animals are *not* kept in small cages. Pastured pork and poultry tend to be richer and meatier than their insipid, flabby counterparts from factory farms. Pastured pork contains more omega-3 fats and vitamin E, and pastured poultry more omega-3 fat and vitamin A, than industrial meat.

Real eggs are pastured, too. Pastured eggs contain significantly more omega-3 fats, which they get from grass and bugs. You can tell a pastured egg right away by the deep yellow yolk, rich in vitamin A from the beta-carotene in grass. The yolks of industrial eggs, by contrast, are pale yellow. Some farmers who don't raise chickens outdoors feed omega-3 fats from fish or flaxseed to hens. One study I've seen shows these eggs are a good source of omega-3 fats, but we don't know what they lack. They must be missing beta-carotene from plants because the chickens don't go outside and the yolks are predictably pale.

*Real meat is free of hormones and antibiotics.* Growth hormones are commonly used in beef cattle to speed weight gain. (Hormones are not permitted in poultry or pig farming.) These hormones are controversial and probably bad for you. When mothers eat a lot of beef during pregnancy, their sons have lower sperm counts and reduced fertility.[10] Researchers suspect that the synthetic hormones in the mother's diet disrupt testicular development in her unborn son, forever compromising his virility.

Antibiotics are also used on cattle, pigs, and chickens to prevent illness from overcrowding and to hasten weight gain. Antibiotic abuse on factory farms has created a major public health problem: drug-resistant bacteria. When the doctors need to treat you for an infection, they have no drug to turn to.

Now you know enough to talk to farmers and read labels intelligently. When shopping for beef and lamb, look for the term

## A QUICK LOOK AT REAL MEAT

| INDUSTRIAL BEEF | ORGANIC BEEF | REAL BEEF |
|---|---|---|
| Corn, grain, and soybeans | Organic grains | Grass and hay |
| Growth hormones | No hormones | No hormones |
| Antibiotics | No antibiotics | No antibiotics |
| Cattle in feedlots | Some "access" to pasture | Cattle graze outside |

### REAL PORK
The best pork is fed organic (or otherwise ecological) corn and other foods, including acorns, coconut, and whey. Pigs are allowed to root freely outdoors, in woods, orchards, or pasture. Heritage breeds raised slowly have more fat and flavor.

### REAL CHICKEN AND EGGS
The best chickens are slow-growing breeds raised on organic (or otherwise ecological) corn and allowed to run free on pasture. They are air-chilled after slaughter. Real eggs have deep yellow yolks from a diet that includes fresh pasture.

"grass fed" on the label. Pork, poultry, and eggs should be "pastured." Organic meat is also a good choice. It will not contain hormones, antibiotics, or pesticides, but it may or may not be grass-fed or pastured.

How meat is handled matters, too. Beef and lamb should be properly aged; that means the butcher hangs it for a while. Industrial chickens are dunked in chlorinated baths, which makes them watery. (You pay for the water.) Air-chilled poultry is best. Look for slow-growing breeds, such as the Naked Neck, which is called *Poulet Rouge Fermier* in the United States. Industrial chickens come to market in five to seven weeks; real chicken is twelve to fourteen weeks old, which makes for deeper flavor and superior texture.

## REAL FISH

People who are thoughtful about food can be fretful about fish. There are genuinely complex questions of nutrition, pollutants, and ecology. There are farmed fish and wild, imported fish and local, not to mention fresh, frozen, and canned. Seafood is the classic example of a knotty personal health and global environmental issue, the kind that makes perfectly intelligent people wail: "Am I supposed to eat fish or not? Which fish?" Don't despair.

Fish or other seafood is vitally important for your health. We've yet to discover a population of humans living for generations without any foods of the sea. In the human diet, fish is a relatively rare source of important omega-3 fats and a great protein if you don't care to eat meat and poultry. It's indispensable for mothers and babies.

Fish are either largely carnivorous (cod, salmon, tuna) or herbivorous (carp, catfish, tilapia). If you're eating carnivores, wild is best. Raising fish whose natural diet is mostly other fish in pens is wasteful; fish farms destroy more fish than they produce. It's also dubious ecologically. Captive salmon sicken wild salmon; shrimp farms destroy mangrove forests. The use of pesticides and antibiotics, mostly to combat conditions caused by overcrowding, is unsavory. Farming fish that are naturally vegetarian is less destructive, but the profits are in carnivores. Organic salmon and shrimp farms are better than factory fish farms, but wild fish from healthy fisheries is best.

Many pregnant women are afraid to eat fish because of methylmercury and fetal brain damage. But we also know that fish is vital for brain growth. The results on this thorny issue are now clear. *Not eating fish poses a greater risk to your baby's brain than eating fish.*

This is what you need to know about fish. The metal mercury is found in the environment. It can combine with carbon to form a toxin called methylmercury. Industrial pollution creates methylmercury, too. Methylmercury is infamous for causing birth defects and brain damage in children. It's no friend of fertility, either. It can cause ovulatory problems, uterine bleeding, and miscarriage. Methylmercury dissolves in water and accumulates up the food chain, which means it's found in higher concentrations in older, bigger, and more carnivorous fish, and it ends up in your tissues when you eat it. If you stop consuming methylmercury, it eventually clears your body.

So if you're pregnant or trying to conceive, eat fish, but not fish high in methylmercury. If you love large fish, such as blue fin tuna, shark, swordfish, and tilefish, you may consume too much. High-grade or "sushi" tuna tends to be high in methylmercury. Good choices are herbivores (catfish, tilapia, freshwater trout), small fish (herring, sardines), smaller, line-caught American tuna, and wild salmon. If you don't eat fish, take a high-quality fish oil.

Real fish is good stuff. Firm, briny, and vibrant with pink and ruby antioxidants, wild salmon tastes strikingly better than farmed salmon, which is greasy, flabby, and bland by comparison. It also contains more omega-3 fats, and fewer pollutants, than farmed salmon. Many would argue that fresh, local seafood

## A QUICK LOOK AT REAL FISH

**Cold-water, oily fish such as sardines and herring have the most omega-3 fats; wild salmon is good, too. Smaller and younger fish contain less methylmercury. Buy smaller, line-caught tuna from American Tuna or Vital Choice. Carnivores (salmon, tuna, shrimp) should be wild. Herbivores (carp, tilapia, catfish, trout) are less destructive when farmed.**

just off the boat is the best eating, and I'm lucky to have superb scallops, bluefish, oysters, and more at local farmers' markets. But with seafood, I'm not a strict locavore. I also buy seafood from the Pacific Coast, three thousand miles away. I happily serve frozen and canned wild Alaskan seafood, including salmon, roe, various white fish, spot prawns, and tuna.

In traditional diets, fish is often raw or lightly cooked. Low heat protects sensitive omega-3 fats from being oxidized, or damaged. Sushi, sashimi, ceviche, smoked salmon, and caviar are among the famous and familiar raw dishes. In Siberia, the Nenet eat stroganina, a kind of sashimi. Instead of peanuts, bar food includes thin, crisp slices of frozen fish that are seasoned with salt and pepper and served with vodka.

## REAL FRUIT AND VEGETABLES

I never have managed to thank my parents properly for my happy childhood amid tomatoes and tomato hornworms, cabbages and cabbage loopers. I was two years old when they started farming, so an abundance of good seasonal vegetables is all I've ever known. It was not an easy life, merely a magical one.

At first, we sold our vegetables by the side of the road in local towns. At eight years old, I found manning roadside stands a lonely business. It wasn't very profitable, either. But we had no other business plan. Then, in 1980, when I was nine, the first farmers' market in our region opened in a parking lot in suburban Arlington, Virginia.

Farming changed my life, and farmers' markets changed it again. It was not long before we gave up roadside stands for good. At market, customers came in droves, and they were crazy about our food. We got to know other farmers and made friends with city dwellers. Life was less isolated, and we ate better. We could buy fresh food we didn't grow ourselves, from peaches to beef. Most of all, the growth of farmers' markets meant we were making money farming.

Happy as I was on the farm, I was equally happy in town, where we were celebrated (it seemed to me) by hordes of grateful eaters. My vegetable luck continues. I live within walking distance of excellent year-round farmers' markets and when my parents, now retired, visit us in New York or at Small Farm, they never fail to bring garden vegetables.

You are lucky too. You don't have to spend your summers picking corn in the cool morning and beans in the hot afternoon, as I did. You don't have to start your own farmers' markets, as I did in London, England, and Washington, D.C., to satisfy my local food addiction. Local food is everywhere.

Don't be intimidated by produce shopping. Just get on with it. The best fruit and vegetables are local, seasonal, and ecological. At a farmers' market with integrity, all the fresh produce must be local and seasonal, but learning about ecological methods takes a little more homework. The ORGANIC, BIODYNAMIC, and CERTIFIED NATURALLY GROWN labels are excellent guides to clean produce (and particularly useful in supermarkets), but you don't have to demand third-party certification when you're shopping directly from the farmer. Just find out whether she uses chemicals or prefers ecological methods.

Research shows that produce grown with natural methods contains fewer chemical residues and more nutrients, including vitamins and antioxidants, than the industrial stuff. That said, I frequently buy local produce from farmers who aren't strictly ecological, and in the winter, I'm a regular in various shops, from supermarkets to the greengrocer, where I often buy imported produce. Here in the Northeast, a girl can get tired of apples and potatoes, and eating fresh fruit and vegetables is just too important for health to make local produce my Holy Grail. Local food is a major consideration, but not the only one.

Superior flavor is the main benefit of eating local and seasonal produce. Having eaten my share of good tomatoes, I often leave the pale red slices you get in industrial food joints untouched. Local food should be fresher, riper, and (yes) often cheaper than the supermarket version, especially when there's a glut. Another benefit of eating local is diversity. Farmers who sell at local markets typically grow more, and more interesting and tasty, varieties than industrial growers. My parents were locally famous for offering a couple of dozen tomatoes and a dozen cucumbers. They did it decades ago, but now it's standard practice.

In vegetables, we seek two main qualities: production (good for farmers) and flavor (good for eaters). Some winners are heirlooms, grown from seeds handed down for generations, while others are hybrids—modern vegetables bred by plant wizards. Both have a warm welcome on good farms and at my table. Hybrids got a bad name from rock-hard, flavorless commercial varieties bred for shipping, but many gardener's varieties, as they're often known, are terrific, and too many heirlooms are simply too pricey. Other heirlooms don't produce well, and some don't even taste good. It's crazy to worship heirlooms, as some foodies do, when there are so many good varieties to eat.

I notice two common mistakes with vegetables. First, people don't buy enough, with predictable results: They don't cook or eat enough vegetables. If your fridge isn't packed with fresh produce, you won't have a couple of vegetables at every meal. I'd rather throw away old vegetables—and often do—than do without at supper time. The same goes for fruit. If the fruit bowl isn't full, your family is not eating fruit.

Second, people worry too much about how to cook vegetables. They're overreliant on recipes, and for some odd reason, dishes must be complicated. You make a list of ingredients, shop, dice, blanch, sauté, make a sauce, bake . . . Who has time for this? I sometimes enjoy these complex, layered numbers in restaurants, but not at home. There is no need to get fancy. I make vegetables at every meal, every day, all year. Here's how:

* Take one vegetable.
* Add one fat and one flavor, or maybe two.
* Salt it.

That's it. The flavor—garlic, fresh herbs, hot peppers—is optional. The fat and salt, however, are not. Most vegetables are low-fat carbohydrates. They are dry and bland, and thus vastly improved by fat (for mouth feel and flavor) and salt, which enhances flavor. So when I cook zucchini, I might choose butter, garlic, and salt. Extra flavor might come from freshly grated Parmigiano Reggiano. Beets I usually dice, roast in olive oil and salt, and then dress with lemon and thyme, maybe tossed with sheep milk feta. For radicchio salad, I'll use olive oil, blue cheese, walnuts, and salt. Cucumber salad with dill, crème fraîche, and salt is ready in minutes. This approach is not only easy to repeat but easy to vary. That's a virtue in home cooking—and in domestic life in general, come to think of it.

You will notice that I didn't invent these combinations. They're all classics from one cuisine or another. Originality is not my goal; eating vegetables is. The only mistake worse than wasting time with fancy recipes is omitting the fat or salt. Omitting both amounts to not cooking. At my table there is no place for naked broccoli. I also think the fashion for al dente vegetables is past its sell-by date. Half-raw green beans, snow peas, and zucchini just don't taste good.

## REAL FATS

I grew up on simple but rich American food, including fried chicken, buttered toast, and granola with nuts and whole milk. My mother believed in real food, especially real fats. That's what she served, and that's what you ate—no whining. I was a happy and healthy kid. But in my teens, I got plump, and by sophomore year I was desperate, as too many girls are, to be thin again. It was the 1980s and the low-fat, high-carbohydrate campaign, allegedly good for your heart and waistline, was in full swing, so, like a typical high achiever, I set about trying to take that advice, and to take it as far as I could.

First I was a vegan, then, to allow myself nonfat yogurt, a vegetarian. I tried nonfat, low-fat, low-saturated fat, and low-cholesterol diets. Of all the faddish diets I tried, I stuck with low-fat the longest, because fat seemed to be the worst villain. When I say "low fat," I mean it. The only fat I would eat was olive oil, and not very much of that. I felt sure this abstemious approach would protect me from heart disease, stroke, breast cancer, and getting fat.

What was my reward for this virtuous diet? I struggled constantly with my weight. I exercised like crazy, I was always hungry, I felt like eating addictively (and often did), and I was often gloomy. Most of all, I was perplexed by women, including my mother, who were thin and yet seemed to eat a lot of rich food, food I wouldn't touch.

I was in my twenties and living in London when I started a string of farmers' markets. Impressed by all the fabulous foods the farmers were bringing—food our customers clearly enjoyed—I began to eat real food again, starting with fish and moving swiftly on to beef, chicken, eggs, butter, and fats of all kinds. It was a pleasant surprise when a host of minor symptoms—such as dry skin and poor digestion—vanished. Some major symptoms, like my winter blues, improved sharply.

But I was utterly astonished when I lost twenty pounds—not overnight, certainly, but effortlessly. In my low-fat days, I ran six miles a day and tortured myself climbing stairs at the gym six days a week. But as I started eating more fat and more protein and less rice and beans, the pounds melted off. At age fifteen, I was a strict nonfat vegetarian and weighed as much as 147 pounds. Now, at age forty-four, I've been 120–125 pounds for many years. I eat more than ever, never skimp on fat, and exercise half as much.

I'm not the only American who was petrified by fat. Nor am I the only American who got fat on nonfat foods. By the way, let me be clear: I was not on a low-fat junk food diet. I ate whole grains, beans, plain yogurt, and a lot of fruit and vegetables. No one challenged my apparently perfect diet. No one knew any better.

Later, I did some homework on real food and learned that the low-fat mantra was wrong. In the last generation, Americans faithfully cut total fat intake from 40 percent of calories to about 33 percent. The result was more weight gain and obesity. What happened? Partly, we ate more food. Which foods? Carbohydrates. From 1971 to 1982, the American food supply served up 3,300 daily calories per capita. By 1997, the food business produced 3,800 calories per person—an extra five hundred calories per day. Ninety percent of the extra calories came from carbohydrates.[11] Not fat. Not protein.

Looking back, I realized that what did me in were nonfat foods like pasta, rice, and juice, plus a notable lack of foods that help keep you trim, like calcium-rich milk, protein, and omega-3 fats in fish. When I eventually understood the nutritional myths that had me snookered and miserable, the biggest headline was that REAL FATS ARE GOOD—even the maligned saturated fats— and its corollary, INDUSTRIAL FATS ARE BAD. It's not complicated. *Eat real fats and avoid industrial ones.*

Natural fats come in three kinds: saturated, monounsaturated, and polyunsaturated. Every food is a blend of these fats, and you need all three for various purposes, from conception to digestion, immunity to thinking. For starters, fats make up cell walls, which regulate the passage of vital materials in and out of cells for every function. The fat types also have unique functions in the body. Polyunsaturated fats from fish are used heavily by the brain. The saturated fats in butter and beef help bones build calcium and keep the digestive tract healthy. Monounsaturated fats in olive oil fight inflammation.

All real fats are healthy in moderation. Moderation implies both balance and quantity. Eat all three kinds of fats, not just one, from lots of different foods. Don't eat too much. How much fat should you eat? I cannot tell you. As with beef, bread, lettuce, chocolate, and any other food, you need to figure out how much fat you need to eat to stay trim and feel good. No one can do it for you.

Industrial fats, on the other hand, are trouble. The first industrial fats to avoid are modern grain and seed oils, such as corn, safflower, sunflower, and soybean oils. The "yellow oils," as I call them, are relatively new in the diet. When Native Americans ate corn oil, they ate it in small quantities, with the whole kernel still intact, including the bran, the fiber, the B vitamins, and the fresh vitamin E. What I'm describing, essentially, is a fresh tortilla made with ground corn, a staple of the traditional diet all over Latin America. Today, corn and soybean oil spouts from the American Midwest like oil from rigs in Texas, and you find cheap oils in all kinds of junk food. Until the 1970s, no humans ate corn oil like we do. As Michael Pollan has written, we are people made of corn.

These polyunsaturated grain and seed oils are not inherently bad. They're trouble because the average American eats far too much of them. They're rich in the omega-6 fat linoleic acid (LA). Like the omega-3 fats, this fat is essential, but in excess, it contributes to obesity, diabetes, heart disease, and cancer. Omega-3 and omega-6 fats should be in balance, but most people eat far too much corn oil and not enough fish oil.

There is no nutritional or culinary reason to eat the yellow oils. You will get all the omega-6 fats you need from traditional foods, such as olive oil, nuts, and whole seeds. Furthermore, most of the yellow oils are pressed and refined under high heat and pressure, which damages the polyunsaturated fats and antioxidant vitamin E, which prevents heart disease and is a natural barrier against spoilage. We don't buy yellow oils or eat foods made with them. We sauté in olive oil and butter.

The other industrial fat to avoid is trans fat, which is created when these same unsaturated, liquid vegetable oils are hydrogenated. In 2002, the National Academy of Sciences said that trans fats have "no known health benefits" and no level of consumption is safe.[12] The average American eats about six grams daily. Once hydrogenated vegetable oils were sold as "heart healthy" alternatives to butter, but it's now clear that trans fats contribute to heart disease in many ways: They lower HDL, raise VLDL, raise lipoprotein (a), which promotes atherosclerosis and clotting, promote inflammation, and reduce blood vessel function.

Trans fats are not pro-baby. According to *The Fertility Diet*, they reduce fertility by increasing inflammation throughout the body, which interferes with ovulation, conception, and early embryonic development. Specifically, trans fats reduce fertility by creating insulin resistance, a common cause of ovulatory disorders. The Nurses' Health Study found that eating just four grams of trans fats daily—about 2 percent of calories if you eat two thousand calories a day—"dramatically" raised the risk of ovulatory infertility. According to the late fats expert Dr. Mary Enig, trans fats also correlate with low birth weight, reduce cream in breast milk, and interfere with the conversion and use of the omega-3 fatty acids docosahexaenoic acid (DHA) and eicosapentaenoic acid (EPA), which build the baby's brain and eyes and help prevent maternal depression.

Trans fats are listed on nutrition labels, so you can avoid them. Just beware of one loophole. If the food contains less than one half a gram of trans fat per serving, the label can declare NO TRANS FAT. But if you eat four servings, you've eaten close to two grams of trans fat. Reading the list of ingredients is more reliable. Don't eat anything containing "hydrogenated" or "partially hydrogenated" fats or oils or "vegetable shortening." Avoid cheap fried foods in fast food spots, where hydrogenated oils are used and reused. The sooner we ban trans fats altogether—as Denmark did in 2003—the better off we'll be.

Meanwhile, stay alert, because the latest industrial fats are already in stores near you. Now that trans fats are known villains, the food industry, ever reluctant to embrace real butter, unveils another man-made fat. The new technology is called interestification. The food industry begins with unsaturated oil and randomly inserts stearic acid (a perfectly good saturated fat in beef and chocolate) into the fatty acids. Next, they scramble the fatty acids, which makes the liquid oil solid, and they can call it TRANS FAT–FREE.

Unfortunately, the evidence so far suggests these fats aren't good for you, either. In a 2007 study comparing naturally saturated palm oil, hydrogenated soybean oil, and interestified soybean oil, K. C. Hayes at Brandeis University found that palm oil—a traditional solid fat for baked goods—was the only fat that didn't alter human metabolism for the worse.[13] The latest industrial fats lower HDL, raise blood sugar, and raise insulin resistance.

Perhaps you've seen an imitation butter made with vegetable oil and "enhanced" with plant sterols to reduce cholesterol. Please avoid this industrial fat, too. Plant sterols are phytoestrogens, and like isoflavones (the estrogens in soy) they disrupt hormones, which can cause infertility and birth defects. Food Standards Australia New Zealand warns that foods containing added plant sterols have not been tested on pregnant or lactating women.

These tales of industrial fats lead me to a sad conclusion. We Americans are not sufficiently skeptical about imitation foods and additives. If you'd rather save your intellectual energy

## A QUICK LOOK AT FATS

### WHAT'S IMPORTANT ABOUT REAL FATS?

- All traditional fats are good for you—no exceptions.
- With animal fats, the diet of the animal matters for our health. Grass is good.
- With vegetable oils, processing damages nutrients. Plant oils should be cold-pressed.

### REAL ANIMAL FATS ARE GOOD

- Fat from grass-fed cattle, sheep, bison, and other game
- Butter and cream from grass-fed cows
- Lard from pastured pigs fed a natural diet
- Poultry fat from pastured chickens, ducks, and geese
- Fish oil (preferably wild), especially cod liver oil

### REAL VEGETABLE OILS ARE GOOD, TOO

- Cold-pressed, extra-virgin olive oil
- Cold-pressed, unrefined flaxseed oil
- Unrefined coconut oil
- Cold-pressed, unrefined macadamia nut, walnut, and sesame seed oils

### WHAT'S WRONG WITH INDUSTRIAL FATS?

- The industrial diet contains too many omega-6 fats from corn and soybean oil, and too few omega-3 fats. This leads to obesity, diabetes, heart disease, and cancer.
- Trans fats cause inflammation, obesity, diabetes, heart disease, and infertility.

### DON'T EAT INDUSTRIAL FATS

- Hydrogenated and partially hydrogenated oils, including lard and vegetable oil
- Interestified fats (vegetable oils made solid but free of trans fats)
- Corn, safflower, sunflower, and soybean oils, especially when refined or heated

for more satisfying and creative work, stop reading the news (good or bad) about the latest industrial food. Don't even look at the fake foods on the shelves. Just buy butter and olive oil, foods with a long history in the human diet. That should simplify your shopping and make time for leisure.


## REAL BREAD

There were not many packaged goods on our shelves when I was growing up. Most everything was made from scratch. Every family member had his nights to cook, plus regular baking chores. Once a week, someone was supposed to make whole wheat bread while someone else made granola with whole oats, nuts, honey, and anything else he wanted to throw in. As I recall, we often ran out of both foods before the scheduled baking day came, especially in the summer. Farmers who work at home tend to snack often. Fresh bread and hot granola quickly disappeared.

My mother, who orchestrated all this, insisted on whole grains. Whole grains naturally contain B vitamins, vitamin E, and fiber. These nutrients are diminished in white flour and white rice. After we bought a small flour grinder, my parents learned to make whole grain pancakes from freshly ground Kamut, brown rice, millet, buckwheat, and other grains. The pancakes are truly delicious, especially studded with local blueberries, hot and runny. Then as now, the only dish in which white flour was always permitted, even encouraged, is in pie crusts, a baking duty Dad has taken over, to family acclaim. ("Chip, you are an artist of pies," said my ten-year-old cousin Nora at our last family reunion.) This deployment of white flour is entirely justified, in my view. Whole wheat crusts crumble every time. And white flour reminds you that even Dad's rhubarb pie is special, not for every day.

Having grown up thinking that bread is the staff of life, and a platform for many great things—such as fresh tomatoes, mayonnaise, and salt—I was taken aback to discover that it is not strictly necessary for health to eat grains or beans at all. We know this because our ancestors, and their prehuman ancestors, had quite a few babies, without any grains and legumes to speak of, for nearly four million years. They did it all with wild game and wild produce. People didn't have grains or beans until about twenty thousand years ago, and they didn't begin to make bread until about eight thousand years ago.

That's right: You don't need oatmeal, rice, or bread at all. The Stone Age diet seems sound nutritionally, and in many ways, it's the way I eat. Winter and summer, our basic supper consists of protein and vegetables. Rob and the children like a piece of toast with butter for breakfast, while most of my starches come from fruit and vegetables. But I can't quite go the whole way. I'm not willing to give up all bread, or rice, lentils, or corn tortillas, to name a few foods we can thank farmers for—not personally, and not as the daily family cook. I like these foods.

Moreover, many people thrive on grains. If you do, there is one thing to understand about grains and legumes and nutrition. They all contain phytic acid, an "antinutrient" which interferes with absorption of protein and of minerals, including calcium, iron, and zinc. In every traditional cuisine, grains and beans are prepared in order to reduce phytic acid and make them more digestible. The main methods of preparation are soaking, fermentation, and sprouting. I usually manage to soak rice, beans, and ground corn overnight, and my mother makes great hot cereal by using oats that have been soaked in whey the previous night.

For bread, the traditional treatment is fermentation, by either a sourdough starter or natural yeast. You can also use flour that has been sprouted. According to Janie Quinn, author of *Essential Eating: The Digestible Diet*, the effect of sprouting is akin to turning hard-to-digest grain into an easily assimilated vegetable. I'm an infrequent baker, so I'm grateful that grains prepared properly are becoming more available. You can buy sprouted-grain flour and breads, and tortillas and tortilla chips made with real nixtamal, just like the Native Americans made them, to reduce phytic acid and get to the vitamin B$_3$.

Unfortunately, real bread and corn chips are not what fills the typical cupboard. Industrial bread and refined grains are everywhere. Jimmy Moore, a blogger who lost 180 pounds by kissing junk carbohydrates good-bye, calls it "carbage." A reader sent me the label from the oxymoronic White Bakery Bread Made With Whole Grain by Sara Lee. The sales pitch is vintage commercial cynicism. "Don't worry, your family will never know that this white bread is good for them." But of course it's not. This junk food masquerading as whole wheat bread contains corn syrup, soy flour, and "natural" flavors.

Carbohydrates account for 50 percent of all calories Americans consume. Fifty percent of those calories come from eight categories of food. In descending order of caloric contribution, they are soft drinks, sodas, and fruit-flavored drinks; cake, sweet rolls, doughnuts, and pastries; pizza; potato chips, corn chips, and popcorn; white rice; bread, rolls, buns, English muffins, and bagels; beer; and French fries and frozen potatoes.

What a list. At least the beer is a traditional fermented food and contains a few B vitamins. These refined carbohydrates are mostly empty calories, meaning they offer little in the way of nutrients. A short list of the missing: fiber, antioxidants, vitamins, minerals. All these foods will cause blood sugar and insulin to spike and plummet, spike and plummet. That makes you insulin resistant and almost certainly fatter. (A few skinny people eat refined carbohydrates and stay skinny. But they don't escape unhealthy insulin levels.)

The Nurses' Health Study found that eating junk carbohydrates is also bad for fertility. Women who ate food with the highest glycemic load—essentially, a measure of refined carbohydrate—were 92 percent more likely to have ovulatory infertility than women with the lowest glycemic load, even accounting for age and smoking. Carbage won't help you get into your "skinny" jeans. It's not good for your heart. Or your ovaries. I could put this message gently, but I don't want to. *Stop eating carbage*.

## REAL FOOD RULES

Recently, journalists, foodists, think-tankers, and the classes who chatter have gotten very excited about local and real food. A favorite story line goes something like this. *This food is great! But it's too expensive. And there are too many choices! People are terribly confused. Is organic better than local or the other way round?* The same story runs again and again. I recommend you don't read these articles. Once you have the information you need about food, there is no correct answer. There is only your taste and your point of view. Here's mine.

*My View on Vegetables*

We were not rich when I was little, but we had all the fresh produce we could eat. From April to November, we grew our own vegetables and ate plenty. What we didn't grow we bought or bartered at the farmers' markets we attended. If we had put a market retail price on our weekly vegetable consumption at Wheatland Vegetable Farms, it would have been way out of proportion to our income. All summer, my parents ate four-dollar-a-pound heirloom tomatoes with abandon. When I visited my parents in their farming years, I'd come home with a trunkful of food: asparagus, Sun Gold cherry tomatoes, Armenian cucumbers, stiff-neck garlic, French crisp lettuce, Romanesco zucchini, Genovese basil. If I were picking up this order of ecological vegetables at any farmers' market, the price would sting.

Winter on the farm was a different matter. In the 1980s, farmers' markets closed in the winter and there were precious few farmers raising local food in heated tunnels, a method common today. But my mother had her convictions, and they included eating fresh fruit and vegetables every day, so off we drove to Magruder's for bargains on large amounts of imported industrial produce. We bought lettuce and red peppers, eggplant and onions. We bought citrus from the annual Future Farmers of America fruit sale. Thus provisioned, we ate a green salad plus vegetables every night; dessert was often apple salad with yogurt and nuts. Even though we have better winter local food now, my mother's philosophy—and mine—hasn't changed. We buy local and ecological when we can and eat vegetables all winter, no matter where we get them.

Good as local, seasonal, and ecological vegetables are, it's more important for your family to eat plenty of fresh fruits and vegetables every day. Lots of studies show that people who eat more fruit and vegetables are healthier than those who don't. I'd bet my last carrot that these studies weren't conducted with local, seasonal, and ecological peas. In deepest winter, when local produce is scarce and expensive here in New York City, I go directly to the supermarket or local greengrocer, head held high, to buy greens. We could live on locally grown lacto-fermented vegetables, but I like fresh vegetables too much. I have no idea what the carbon footprint of these choices is.

It's also possible to avoid most pesticides if you're willing to shop selectively. Using government data from fifty-one thousand tests, the Environmental Working Group determined the most contaminated and the cleanest produce. They reckon you can reduce pesticide exposure substantially by eating the Clean Fifteen instead of the Dirty Dozen. Get the latest list at www .FoodNews.org.

## The Food Chain Principle

You'll recall that fat-soluble pesticides and other toxins climb up the food chain and gather there. If the steer was fattened on a feedlot, the pesticide residue from many bushels of corn and soy is concentrated in the fat of the steak. The methylmercury in fish is more concentrated in larger, older fish. There are more fat-soluble hormones in a pat of butter than in a relatively watery glass of milk. So the higher up the food chain I'm shopping, the more I'll spend to get clean food.

I think of our food budget as a top-heavy pyramid. At the bottom are large volumes of "light" and relatively inexpensive produce. I mean light in weight (lettuce) or nutrients (a cucumber is mostly water). I buy produce every couple of days, by the bagful, and every night we eat a salad and a couple of cooked vegetables. At the farmers' market, I buy equally from the ecological and the not-so-ecological farmers. We could afford to spend more for organic produce every time without feeling the pinch, but I don't.

At the top of our pyramid are foods at the top of the food chain: physically and nutritionally dense animal protein, dairy, eggs, and fats. We eat these foods every day, and we are not stingy about quantity. I am always willing to spend relatively more (per pound, per dozen) to buy grass-fed, pastured, and drug-free beef, pork, poultry, milk, cheese, and eggs. The same is true of fats. We buy good butter with high fat content, unrefined, organic coconut oil, and extra-virgin olive oil, even for frying.

When shopping high on the food chain, I make two other distinctions. First, I make a bigger effort. I've spent years looking for the best milk in our region. We can choose from a handful of good local grass-fed milks. At last I found shrimp I'm happy with: wild Pacific spot prawns from Vital Choice and farmed Pacific White shrimp from Ecofarms. Second, I'm more willing to leave the region to shop. There's no good olive oil nearby, so we look to California and Chile. Third, I choose different meats for different recipes. Frozen grass-fed local beef makes nice bolognese, meatloaf, and chili, but for burgers we like it freshly ground and I cannot always find it grass-fed. If we can't get a good local rib eye or pork roast, we buy it from a national brand with high standards. We don't buy local food to occupy what the marketing people call the "virtue position." We eat local food because it tastes better.

*Stop Counting*

The title of a 2007 article in *Nutrition Reviews* puts it squarely: "Food, Not Nutrients, Is the Fundamental Unit in Nutrition."[14] The piece declares that whole foods have complex effects and that the narrow focus on nutrients has obscured the value of eating real food. Worse, it's been harmful. The authors call for nutrition researchers to "think food first." How radical.

We've fallen prey to a reductive and counterproductive approach. The Australian sociologist Gyorgy Scrinis called it "nutritionism," and Michael Pollan made it famous in his wonderful book *In Defense of Food*. "Nutritionism" is a state of mind. Under its sway, we think of nutrients (lycopene) instead of food (tomato). Pollan dates "The Age of Nutritionism" to a 1982 report called *Diet, Nutrition, and Cancer*. Each chapter focused on a single nutrient. Writes Pollan,

> The National Academy of Sciences report helped codify the official new dietary language, the one we all still speak. Industry and media soon followed suit, and terms like *polyunsaturated, cholesterol, monounsaturated, carbohydrate, fiber, polyphenols, amino acids, flavanols, carotenoids, antioxidants, probiotics,* and *phytochemicals* soon colonized much of the cultural space previously occupied by the tangible material formerly known as food.

Nutritionism has been good for the food companies and supplement sellers ready to profit from government-approved health claims. Orange juice with added calcium and chocolate with added probiotics would not exist if not for the nearly universal acceptance of nutritionism. But it has not been noticeably good for our health.

The alert reader will now sniff a paradox. Nutritionism hasn't served us well, and like the sensible Michael Pollan, I'm against it. Yet the book in your hands, like my last book, is fortified and enriched with facts and arguments one could justifiably describe as nutritionist. Far better if I confess now. I'll talk about the nutrients you need in order to have a healthy baby and where to get them. I don't know a better way.

However, I don't live under the banner of nutritionism. I don't count calories, grams of saturated fat, milligrams of vitamin E, micrograms of folic acid, or jillibeters of anything else. It would be downright wacky to create shopping lists of nutrients. ("I'm pregnant! Don't forget complex carbohydrates, lauric acid, and betaine.") As a nutrition geek, I have a basic understanding of the major nutrients and a few minor ones, but I am still firmly in favor of the tangible material formerly known as food. In our house we call it real food. It's good for you. It's good for babies. It's good for everybody.

## CHAPTER 2

# The Fertility Diet

### TRADITIONAL FERTILITY FOODS

When I decided to try to have a baby, I went to the nurse-midwife with questions. I'd been taking the birth control pill. Should we wait a bit before trying? Did we need blood tests, or screening for genetic diseases? But my main question was about food. What should I eat? What should Rob eat? "No one has ever come to me for preconception counseling on diet," she said. "Good for you."

I confess we had tried baby-making a few times before I got to the midwife. I'm not that organized. But I wasn't smug on hearing that most couples don't think of eating to conceive; I was surprised. I take for granted that good nutrition affects every part of the body. It hadn't occurred to me to embark on pregnancy *without* expert advice.

Not so long ago, mothers, grandmothers, aunts, and various busybodies would have offered these services to newlyweds as a matter of course. In traditional cultures, young couples were expected to conceive within weeks or months of getting hitched. The *Caraka Samhita*, the Sanskrit text of traditional Ayurvedic medicine, contains long chapters on fertility and conception. But modern American pregnancy culture has little to say about eating *before* you're eating for two. Bossy as modern nutritionists are about avoiding whole milk—and everything else that used to be considered good—I think they've dropped the ball on the fertility diet.

Eating well before you try to get pregnant serves two purposes. It helps you conceive, and it helps you have a healthy baby. Vitamin E, for example, is a powerful fertility nutrient. Fat-soluble vitamin E was first called "Fertility Factor X" in 1922 because animals cannot reproduce without it. The pituitary gland, the body's master regulator of hormones, requires vitamin E. Vitamin E is essential for sperm production; severe deficiency can cause permanent sterility. But don't panic. If you eat olive oil, nuts, avocados, and whole grains, you and your baby's father will get plenty of vitamin E.

Even at the moment of conception, diet matters. The right foods put the baby on the right track for life. There is some evidence that a mother's nutritional health at the time of *conception* has more influence on birth weight than her nutrition during pregnancy.[1] If malnutrition is severe, embryonic development and DNA replication may be damaged in ways that cannot be corrected later.

Once you're pregnant, there are many good things you can do for yourself and your baby. Getting more sleep is one. But good food is the sine qua non of a healthy pregnancy. You will build six or eight pounds of brand-new baby from your own flesh and blood. Right from the start, eating well will support a healthy placenta, which will be the baby's only means of getting nutrients and oxygen. Next, a steady supply of good food ensures the baby will develop properly, grow well, and gain weight. A healthy birth weight starts a healthy life. Low birth weight is linked to adult health problems, including low bone density, high blood pressure, Type 2 diabetes, and heart disease.[2]

Your diet can even affect your baby's genes in the womb. Certain nutrients, or lack of them, can turn genes on or off, without changing the DNA itself. This, in turn, affects the baby's chances of, say, being obese or getting cancer.[3] The groundbreaking experiment in gene expression involved fat mice with "fat" genes.[4] Researchers fed fat-gene pregnant mice B vitamins, including folic acid, $B_{12}$, choline, and betaine. To everyone's surprise, the well-fed pregnant mice gave birth to thin babies, not fat ones—even though they inherited "fat" genes from their mothers, and even though they were genetically identical to the fat babies of fat-gene mothers who didn't get vitamins. In other words, in the topsy-turvy world of epigenetics, the right nutrients can make "fat" genes act like "thin" ones. Geneticists were startled by this finding, which appeared to contradict a fundamental Darwinian principle—that environment cannot change inheritance. But it can. Today epigenetics is exploding with similar findings on the needs of mothers and babies.

Official government advice and conventional wisdom, however, are still in the Dark Ages. I was heartened to see that the Centers for Disease Control started a campaign on "Preconception Care" to encourage fertile women to prevent health problems for mother and baby before they conceive. The guidelines are simple and affordable. They include screening for sexually transmitted diseases, treating diabetes, switching to baby-friendly medications, getting certain vaccinations, and losing excess weight. Each is proven to prevent a known health problem in mother or baby. I've no doubt this public health initiative will be cost-effective if it succeeds.

Still, I couldn't help but notice that only one of the fourteen recommendations for preconception care is about food. Actually, it's about a synthetic nutrient. Like other experts, the CDC advises women of child-bearing age to take synthetic folic acid, which prevents neural tube defects such as spina bifida and anencephaly—often before you know you're pregnant—by an astonishing 60 percent. This is good advice. It seems that some women don't get enough natural folate from foods like chicken, fish, leafy greens, fruit, nuts, and lentils. There are few defects so tragic as spina bifida and few preventive measures so effective as supplements. We are lucky folic acid is affordable and available. But there is so much more to making healthy babies.

Compare our modern, reductive approach with traditional cultures, where many special foods were reserved for newlyweds,

## EATING TO CONCEIVE = EATING FOR TWO

**We'll talk about fertility first, but the fertility diet is not markedly different from the pregnancy diet. That's largely because good food is good food, plain and simple. It's also because conception rolls rapidly into pregnancy. The same foods that help you conceive will, mere days later, help keep the rapidly growing embryo healthy. The fine line between conception and pregnancy is apparent when you ponder the heartbreaking case of early miscarriage. Vitamin E, for example, helps you conceive, and it helps prevent miscarriage. With a few variations, mother and baby need the same good foods from conception to two years, and after age two, children may eat all the good real foods adults do.**

always with babies in mind. Foods considered essential included butter, liver, egg yolks, and seafood, especially fish liver and eggs. We know about these fertility foods from Weston Price, a dentist who traveled the world studying traditional diets in the 1930s. Price collected his anthropological studies and lab work in a classic work, *Nutrition and Physical Degeneration*, six hundred data-dense pages on what people ate before white flour, sugar, refined vegetable oil, and other junk food wrecked their health in just one or two generations.[5] Although he was initially interested in teeth, Price also studied general health, and he was struck by the attention paid to mothers. "Many primitive people have understood the necessity for special foods before marriage, during gestation, during the nursing period and for rebuilding before the next pregnancy," he wrote.

Dairy and seafood were prominent fertility foods in traditional diets. Together they offer four vital nutrients, without which a woman simply cannot get pregnant: vitamins A and D, iodine, and omega-3 fats. Real dairy provides all four, especially the fat-soluble vitamins. Among the herding Maasai in Kenya, "girls were required to wait for marriage until the time of the year when the cows were on the rapidly growing green grass and to use the milk from these cows for a certain number of months before they could be married," wrote Price. In Swiss villages, Price found, the fertility diet featured spring-grass butter. As you see, the Swiss and Maasai drank real milk. It's demonstrably superior to modern milk. Lush-season Maasai milk contains more fat, choline, and cholesterol—all good baby foods—than modern industrial milk.[6]

Seafood is a traditional fertility food for its precious omega-3 fats and iodine, as well as vitamins $B_{12}$ and D. As with spring-grass butter, people went to a lot of trouble for seafood. Peruvian tribes high in the Andes, far away from water, traveled hundreds of miles to trade with valley tribes for kelp and roe. "Fish eggs were an important part of the nutrition of the women during their reproductive period," wrote Price. "They were available both at

## FOOD AND SEX

When I picked up *The Orgasmic Diet*, I was skeptical. Marenna Lindberg is almost comically orgasmic—after she changes her diet to real food, of course. Happily, there's little sex in this book and plenty of sound nutrition for a healthy sex life. Women need testosterone, the hormone of desire; balanced dopamine and serotonin levels; and good circulation. Eating good protein, real fat, whole grains, dark chocolate, and fish will keep hormones and circulation healthy. Steer clear of white flour and sugar, trans fats, caffeine, cigarettes, and the pill. Men and women should avoid vegan and low-fat diets and industrial soy foods, which kill testosterone. "A little soy here and there . . . won't have much of an impact on your sex life," writes Lindberg. "But if you are constantly eating meal replacement bars and tofu and drinking soy milk, just say no. Embrace real foods." Instead of soy, she recommends meat, eggs, milk, cheese, and nuts. Arousal in men depends on nitric oxide for blood vessel dilation. The body makes it from the amino acid arginine. Eating fresh spinach, crustaceans, fish, turkey, oats, almonds, and walnuts keeps nitric oxide flowing. Men also need zinc and iron, which makes beef an excellent sex food.

the coast market of Peru and as dried fish eggs in the highland markets, whence they were obtained by the women in the high Sierras to reinforce their fertility and efficiency for childbearing." Even Eskimos in Alaska—who virtually lived on fish and would seem to have all the necessary omega-3 fats and iodine— ate dried fish eggs for fertility.

In traditional cultures, eating for two was a village affair. In the Fiji islands of the Pacific, the tribal leader called a community meal to celebrate each pregnancy. "At this feast the chief appointed one or two young men to be responsible for going to the sea from day to day to secure the special seafoods that expectant mothers need to nourish the child," wrote Price. In his lab, Price found that the large, spidery crabs the boys fetched for pregnant women were high in vitamins A and D.

## FOUR FERTILITY RULES

Traditional diets are fascinating. Stories about what people eat and why could fill many books—and have. But it's not necessary to understand every detail or even to eat exactly as traditional people do. You merely need to get the nutrients they knew they needed. Here's what I've learned about food and fertility from time-honored diets.

### 1. Be an Omnivore

Make no mistake. The high-status fertility foods in traditional diets are largely of animal origin. That's not to diminish spinach, nuts, oranges, or olive oil. All these are good foods, and you can be sure that most traditional diets contained plenty of fresh plants. But it's difficult to get pregnant and build a robust baby on a diet of plant foods alone. That's probably why there are no long-standing, strictly vegan societies. There are groups of modern vegans all over the world, of course. Many Jains, a religious sect in India, eat a vegan diet, although it's not compulsory. But anthropologists have yet to identify a society living on plant foods alone, without synthetic supplements, spanning generations of vegan mothers and fathers, children and grandchildren.

Price hoped to find one. After visiting Vitu Levu, a large island in the Pacific Ocean, he wrote, "One of the purposes of the expedition to the South Seas was to find, if possible, plants or fruits which together, without the use of animal products, were capable of providing all of the requirements for growth and for maintenance of good health." No luck. "I have not found a single group . . . building and maintaining excellent bodies by living entirely on plant foods." Instead, he saw people seeking foods of animal origin for special cases, such as fertility. In Africa, for example, the largely vegetarian Kikuyu tribe fed girls on a special diet containing extra animal fat for six months before marriage.

People often ask if I'm aware that the Academy of Nutrition and Dietetics says that vegan diets are "appropriate" for pregnancy, lactation, and in infancy. I am. But I've read the 2009 Position Paper of the Academy (formerly American Dietetic Association) and I find the evidence cited unsatisfactory. For example, the Academy researchers found no studies on birth outcomes (length, weight) for vegan pregnancy.

Even the Academy authors note that a vegan diet presents challenges for fertility and pregnancy because several key nutrients are missing, or missing in sufficient quantity, from plants. Vitamin $B_{12}$ is found only in animal products. According to the Vegetarian Society, humans cannot use the plant form of $B_{12}$. And according to the Academy, not even fermented soy sauce contains adequate active vitamin $B_{12}$. Women with low $B_{12}$ have more babies with spina bifida.[7] Vegans who do not take synthetic vitamin $B_{12}$ risk having babies with nerve disorders. Iron may be lacking on a vegan diet because the iron from plants is poorly absorbed. Eggs need a supply of iron to make proteins and DNA.[8] So do sperm. Iron raises sperm counts. The best iron comes from red meat and liver.

A vegan diet lacks fully formed DHA and EPA. These vital omega-3 fats are found only in fish and in small quantities in grass-fed meat, dairy, and eggs. Studies show that vegetarians and vegans have significantly lower levels of EPA and DHA.[9] One study found that vegan EPA levels were 22 percent of those of omnivores and DHA levels 38 percent of those of omnivores. Although your body can make some of these omega-3 fats from related fats in flaxseed and walnuts, the conversion is slow and uncertain. Sperm is rich in DHA.

Getting complete protein is another challenge for vegans. Only animal foods contain all the amino acids essential for human life in the right proportions. Soy, for example, lacks adequate methionine, and corn lacks adequate lysine and tryptophan. Protein from meat, fish, poultry, dairy, and eggs is superior in quantity and quality to any plant protein.

Egg production, sperm count, and sperm motility depend on adequate protein. You cannot make luteinizing hormone (LH) and

## PERFECT PROTEIN

Because amino acid composition in high-quality protein varies, what is considered "perfect" is arbitrary. Experts have chosen the egg to represent the ideal combination of amino acids for human health. An equally valid approach is to consider human milk the ideal protein. With breast milk at the top, these are the relative protein quality ratings for various foods.[10]

| | |
|---|---|
| Breast milk | 100 |
| Egg | 94 |
| Cow milk | 84 |
| Fish | 83 |
| Meat | 74 |
| Soybeans | 73 |
| Corn | 60 |

follicle stimulating hormone (FSH), the hormones that prompt the egg to mature, without it. Two small studies suggest protein aids fertility in women.[11] Nonmenstruating athletes tend to eat less protein than menstruating athletes. Another study comparing meat eaters and vegetarians found that the vegetarians had more ovulatory problems.

Don't rely on soy for protein if you're hoping to conceive. Soy phytoestrogens alter the menstrual cycle, change hormone levels, and even stop ovulation. The doses causing these problems are not large. Eating thirty grams of pickled soybeans[12] or sixty grams of soy protein will disrupt menstrual cycles.[13] One soy estrogen, genistein, is toxic to the thyroid, which also reduces fertility. "There is abundant evidence that some of the isoflavones found in soy . . . demonstrate toxicity in estrogen-sensitive tissues and in the thyroid," wrote two FDA experts. "No dose is without risk."[14]

If you do eat soy, eat traditional soy foods, such as tofu, in moderation. The best soy foods are fermented, such as miso and natto. Phytic acid in unfermented soy blocks nutrients, including protein, calcium, and zinc. Don't eat any industrial soy products made with isolated soy protein. They contain far too many plant estrogens. Don't eat imitation foods made with soy protein, such as soy "milk" or "burgers."

Many traditional cultures, from Asia to India, are largely vegetarian. The difference between a vegan and a vegetarian diet is dairy and eggs. Even if you never touch meat, fish, or poultry, eating either milk products or eggs will cover the main fertility nutrients. Dairy or eggs will provide complete protein, vitamin $B_{12}$, vitamins A and D, and even a few omega-3 fats if the milk is grass fed and the eggs are pastured. If you don't eat seafood, add unrefined sea salt and sea vegetables for iodine. Small quantities of these foods can make a big difference. Practitioners who treat infertility have told me that infertile vegans conceive after starting to eat a little fish, dairy, or eggs.

However, please note: Once you're pregnant, your baby needs fish oil. A dedicated vegetarian could take unrefined

## FERTILITY AWARENESS

Fertility Awareness (FA) is a natural method of birth control and a fertility aid. You watch and note some simple body signs, learn a few rules of interpretation, and then you know on which days you can get pregnant. Couples who use FA love it. Your FA chart can tell you if your cycle is regular or hint at why you're not getting pregnant. According to Katie Singer, author of *The Garden of Fertility,* poor diet can cause ovulatory infertility. Women with irregular cycles often eat too many refined carbohydrates and too much soy protein. "Their diets often lack nutrient-dense foods and may be vegan or low fat," Singer writes. The charts of vegan women often indicate thyroid problems or failure to ovulate. Many women ovulate again after cutting out soy or sugar and eating cod liver oil, butter, and eggs for essential vitamins A and D.

flaxseed or walnut oil and hope her body converts enough of it to DHA and EPA, but I don't recommend it. It's traditional—and more reliable—to get it directly from fish.

2. *Fat and Fertility*
Spared the temptations of corn syrup and corn chips, our distant ancestors were mostly lean, but plump figures were not unknown. We know this partly from delightful Venus figurines, common artifacts of early human history carved or chipped from ivory, stone, and bone. Many fat goddesses were left by hunter-gatherer societies in Europe and Asia in the final days of the last Ice Age, about ten thousand to thirty thousand years ago. These little women have large hips, bottoms, and thighs for a reason. Fat is closely linked to femininity, motherhood, and fertility. The features of Venus girls may be exaggerated, but the human body hasn't changed much. Fat still counts.

So it's no surprise that traditional fertility foods either *are* fats (butter) or contain plenty (eggs, liver, crab). Village elders don't assign teenage boys to gather wheat and barley for pregnant women. They send them off for fatty seafood. I've yet to find a traditional fertility, pregnancy, or nursing diet that limits fats in any way. In India, butter and ghee are recommended for easy childbirth. Ghee is clarified butter, which means the protein, carbohydrate, and water have been removed, leaving pure butterfat. A rich Indian drink—milk with almonds and saffron—is said to ensure the proper development of the baby, and no wonder. It's crammed with fertility nutrients. In addition to omega-3 fats (if the milk is from grass-fed cows), this drink contains all the fat-soluble vitamins: A, D, E, and $K_2$.

Fertility foods include fats partly because certain fats, such as omega-3 fats in fish, are essential for human health. You cannot live without them. Fats also carry notable fertility nutrients, such as vitamin A, which you need to make estrogen. In his lab, Price found the main fertility foods—shellfish, organ meats, spring butter—extremely rich in three fat-soluble vitamins: A, D, and a mystery ingredient he called Activator X. Researchers now believe this is vitamin $K_2$, which is essential for healthy bones and infant growth.

Fat-soluble vitamins are found in fats for the simple reason that you need fat to digest them. You also need fat to absorb antioxidants such as beta-carotene (in carrots, red peppers, and sweet potatoes) and lycopene (in tomatoes). A salad with fat-free dressing provides scarcely any antioxidants, which are important for sperm health.[15] Much of nutrition comes down to availability rather than quantity. You can eat all the beta-carotene and vitamin A you want, but if you don't eat fats, it won't do any good.

### 3. The Seafood Principle

*Homo sapiens* is unusual in several ways. Unlike the apes, we are hairless, we carry fat under our skin, and we walk on two legs. Compared to our primate cousins, we have enormous brains. And we love the water. Pregnant and laboring women are drawn to water. Until he is four months old, a newborn can hold his breath under water. According to a magnificent book by the obstetrician Michel Odent, *We Are All Water Babies*, every baby is born with the "diving reflex." Even our chemistry is watery. Human blood and tears are salty, like the sea.

In these and other ways, we resemble aquatic mammals more than gorillas, chimps, and monkeys, and that's why the marine biologist Sir Alister Hardy called us the Aquatic Ape. The Aquatic Ape has a strong urge to live near streams, rivers, and oceans—or, failing that, to trade with people who do. The reason is simple. Humans cannot get by—and women cannot get pregnant—without nutrients found chiefly in the sea. They are the omega-3 fats and iodine.

The link between iodine and babies is easy to explain. Hypothyroidism is a common and reversible cause of miscarriage and unexplained infertility, and iodine prevents it. Iodine is found in seafood, including kelp, fish, roe, and milt (fish sperm). We need iodine in only tiny amounts. People who can't get fish are creative about finding iodine. In Africa, tribes cooked with the burned ashes of certain plants to get it. In North America, Indians ate the iodine-rich thyroid glands of male moose for fertility. Butter and eggs can provide adequate iodine, too. You need vitamin A to absorb it.

Seafood is the only food source of the omega-3 fat DHA. DHA is found in high concentrations in sperm. Some men with unexplained infertility have low levels of seminal prostaglandins, which are made from omega-3 fats. Fish oil encourages blood flow to the uterus and reduces certain immune cells called "natural killers," which can affect embryo implantation. DHA is indispensable during pregnancy. The fish-eating ways of *Homo sapiens* are thought to account for our very large brain at birth.

Today, it's easy to take DHA and iodine for granted, but for most of human history, they were hard to come by. You had to live near the sea to get them. In the early twentieth century, a goiter epidemic struck Americans living where the soil was

## MERCURY FILLINGS AND FERTILITY

**Perhaps you have silver amalgam fillings. They contain elemental mercury. Once it was thought that mercury was bound up in fillings, but now it's understood that fillings leak, and thanks to activists like Moms Against Mercury, the FDA finally admitted that "dental amalgams contain mercury, which may have neurotoxic effects on the nervous systems of developing children and fetus." Norway and Sweden banned mercury fillings entirely. If you can, replace mercury fillings with gold or porcelain before you try to conceive. *Never have fillings removed while pregnant or nursing.* Mercury vapor released by drilling seeps into your blood and breast milk.**

iodine-poor. That's why table salt contains iodine by law. But I never buy it. Iodized salt has prevented goiter, but it hasn't cured thyroid disorders, a major cause of infertility. I only use unrefined sea salt, which contains ample natural iodine and a host of other essential trace minerals.

### 4. Don't Eat Carbage

In eastern Australia, Price found that the birth rate among whites had dropped so fast that "many families had no children and many women could produce only one child." Politicians were distressed. On August 1, 1938, the Associated Press reported that the New South Wales Legislature had proposed a "stork derby," with prizes, to boost the falling birth rate. Price suspected junk food was causing infertility. The local diet consisted largely of "refined white-flour products, sugar, polished rice, [refined] vegetable fats, canned goods and a limited amount of meat." This menu of industrial foods was nothing like the whole foods Australian Aborigines ate.

Refined foods are not pro-baby. They lack B vitamins and vitamin E, which are lost when whole grains become white flour. You need both to conceive. Another reason to eat whole foods is that many nutrients work together. Sperm health improves dramatically when vitamins A and E are eaten together, probably because E prevents oxidation of A. You need vitamin C to absorb iron, and saturated fats extend the use of omega-3 fats. There are countless relationships like this in nutrition. There is no need to remember them. Just eat whole foods in their natural state and in classic combinations, such as leaves with olive oil, or fish with butter, and you'll get everything you need.

A second reason to avoid refined foods is insulin resistance, which causes a cascade of hormonal disruptions. When you eat refined carbohydrates instead of fat, protein, and whole grains, cells are overexposed to sugar and to insulin, which spikes when you eat sugar. The cells become "insulin resistant," or deaf to insulin. The usual result is weight gain. Insulin resistance also raises testosterone, which interferes with egg production; promotes insulin-like growth factors, which inhibit FSH; and causes the pituitary gland to make too much LH. All these symptoms plague women with polycystic ovary syndrome (PCOS), the most common cause of ovulatory infertility. Women with PCOS have irregular or absent periods, excess facial and body hair, and enlarged ovaries with small cysts. The cysts are immature eggs; they never mature.

## GOING OFF THE PILL

**Many healthy women can get pregnant soon after stopping the pill. According to *Conceive* magazine, most women get their first postpill period in four to six weeks, 80 percent will be ovulating by three months, and 95 percent within the year. It's probably wise to let your hormones settle down before trying to get pregnant. You can conceive as soon as you ovulate, of course, but you might want to replenish your body first. The pill depletes fertility and pregnancy nutrients, including folate, vitamins A, $B_6$, and C, and zinc.**

To treat infertility caused by PCOS, you must first tackle insulin resistance. Don't eat sugar, white flour, or white rice. When you snack, try chicken, nuts, celery, or fruit. Eat whole grains, and every time you eat any carbohydrate, have some fat or protein, such as butter or cheese, too. Losing 5 to 10 percent of your weight can also help you get pregnant.[16] If you don't have PCOS, but you're overweight, the same advice applies. Eat whole foods and lose a little weight. High blood sugar and insulin resistance—even without a full-blown case of PCOS—also impair fertility.[17]

## THE MODERN FERTILITY DIET

Perhaps the wanderings and writings of Dr. Weston Price seem distant or irrelevant to you. I know you're not living on white rice and canned foods in the New South Wales of the 1930s. I know you're not likely to find moose thyroid in wine sauce in a local restaurant. That's not the point. The point is to absorb the lessons of his pioneering studies. Dr. Thomas Cowan, a family doctor in California, treats infertility with food. "The diet is a whole program," he says. "It means cutting out sugar, chips, and white flour products. It means eating whole foods—including organic meat and animal fats, free-range eggs, fresh vegetables, and soaked grains; and supplementing with cod liver oil. I've seen women on the diet improve or reverse everything from PMS to anovulation, polycystic ovary syndrome, hypothyroidism, endometriosis, menopause problems, and inability to conceive or carry a pregnancy to term."[18]

If you're ready to have a baby, change your diet first. Much of what makes you fertile (such as estrogen) or not (such as trans fats) lodges in your fat. Eating real food will replace and replenish the nutrients in your tissues, but this takes time. If you've eaten a poor diet for years, it might be worth losing a little weight and replacing it with new weight from good foods for a couple of months.

Meanwhile, if you're unsure about your diet, a basic prenatal vitamin provides a little insurance. Women taking a multivitamin conceive more readily than those who don't, and have more twins, too.[19] Folic acid and iron are two ingredients in most prenatal supplements that seem to improve ovulatory infertility. Some women take up to eight hundred micrograms of folic acid, twice the dose often recommended, to aid conception and prevent birth defects. That's The Nurses' Health Study found that at least seven hundred micrograms of folic acid improves ovulation and conception.[20] If you eat plenty of real food, that's probably all you need to do. If you don't, I suggest a little cod liver oil, for vitamins A and D. If you're surprised to find yourself pregnant, don't fret. Just start eating well. Most mothers and babies do just fine.

My own fertility diet was basic. I took extra folic acid and a little cod liver oil. I always eat a lot of wild salmon, but it was midwinter, so I happened to be taking fish oil and B vitamins to prevent the seasonal gloom I used to know well. Here and there, my diary says "bison heart" or some other obscure traditional food, but I can assure you those meals were rare. Most American

## CAFFEINE, ALCOHOL, AND FERTILITY

Too much caffeine is not good for fertility, but no one knows exactly how much is too much.[21] Most experts agree that excess caffeine is not baby-friendly. Miscarriage is twice as likely when women drink two hundred milligrams or more caffeine daily.[22] A sensible (but not ironclad) daily upper limit for caffeine is two cups of coffee or six cups of tea. Two ounces of 70-percent chocolate contains about 80 milligrams of caffeine. Studies on the effects of drinking alcohol on fertility are also mixed. At least one suggests it helps, some say it hurts, and others find no effect.[23] Light drinking is probably fine; we lack definitive evidence about moderate drinking. Heavy drinking is not good for mother or child.

women get pregnant without eating bison heart. I drank a glass of wine at dinner, as I usually did, in those days. Otherwise, I ate my normal diet of real food.

On Valentine's Day, I saw the chiropractor and happened to mention that my period was due. Dr. Steve Macagnone, who has uncommonly sensitive hands and a sensitive mind too, gently explored the familiar bumps at the back of my head, on either side of my neck. "I don't think so, Nina. I think you're pregnant." Less than an hour later, I was at home, peeing on a stick. The stick said yes.

## FIVE EASY PIECES

Eating to conceive is easy. You can cover all the fertility nutrients with just *five good foods*. For vitamins A, D, and K₂, drink *whole milk*. For vitamin E, be generous with extra-virgin *olive oil*. For folate, have a *green salad*. For iodine, eat *wild salmon* or any seafood. For zinc and vitamin B₁₂, *any red meat* will do. It's just plain real food—and substituting other real foods is fine. If you don't like milk, eat cheese instead. If you don't like salmon, try tuna. If you forget what to eat or why, consult the accompanying chart, and if you suspect you're not getting enough real food, consider a supplement.

### More on Vitamin A

You cannot make estrogen without vitamin A. Deficiency is associated with difficult periods, fibroids, and endometriosis.[24] Men need it too. The Sertoli cells, which house and nurture immature sperm, use a lot of vitamin A. In early pregnancy, adequate vitamin A should really be considered as important as folate. Differentiation of cells, the key activity of the new embryo, depends on it. The need for vitamin A begins when the primitive heart and circulation and hindbrain begin to form. That's about week two or three, often before you know you're pregnant.[25]

## FERTILITY NUTRIENTS FOR WOMEN

|  | BENEFITS | BEST FOODS | PILLS, ETC. |
|---|---|---|---|
| Folate | Conception Spinal cord | Liver, leaves, lentils, nuts, chicken | Brewer's yeast |
| Iodine | Healthy thyroid | Fish, roe, kelp, unrefined sea salt | Kelp tablets |
| Iron | Protein, DNA | Red meat, liver | Brewer's yeast, Floradix |
| Vitamin A | Estrogen Organs | Butter, eggs | Cod liver oil |
| Vitamin $B_{12}$ | Conception Prevents spina bifida | Meat, poultry, fish, clams, milk, eggs | Vitamin $B_{12}$ |
| Vitamin D | Sex hormones Organs | Milk, pork, seafood | Cod liver oil |
| Vitamin E | Healthy placenta Oxygen to baby | Olive oil, nuts | Vitamin E |
| Vitamin $K_2$ | Infant growth Healthy bones Healthy sperm | Goose liver, cheese, natto, butter, eggs | Butter oil |
| Zinc | Sperm and eggs Cell division Healthy thyroid | Oysters, beef, shrimp | Brewer's yeast |

True vitamin A is found only in animal foods, including butter, eggs, and liver. The "vitamin A" in carrots and other orange vegetables is actually a precursor, beta-carotene, which the body must convert to usable vitamin A. But that conversion is uncertain, so it's wise to get true vitamin A from animal foods. When you do eat vegetables, a good way to get more beta-carotene is to eat them with fat. Making vitamin A requires bile salts produced by the liver, and bile is in short supply after a low-fat meal. Just add olive oil to salads and butter your sweet potatoes.

### More on Vitamin D

Men and women also need vitamin D to make sex hormones. Deficiency is associated with menstrual cramps, polycystic ovary syndrome, premenstrual syndrome, and infertility.[26] Like vitamin A, vitamin D helps regulate cell growth and differentiation, the process that determines what a cell is to become and begins from the moment of conception. Vitamin D deficiencies are coming back. Dr. Michael Holick of the Department of Medicine at Boston University Medical Center says 40 to 100 percent of American women have marginal vitamin D status.[27] Foods are the best source of vitamin D, but it seems most people don't get enough, perhaps because herring, pork, and cod liver oil are not in fashion.

Get some sun, too. Your body can manufacture vitamin D from cholesterol if your skin is exposed to sunlight. People most at risk of vitamin D deficiency have dark skin, keep their skin covered in public, live in northern climates, and spend their midday hours indoors. Getting twenty minutes of sunlight on as much skin as you can expose, even in the dead of winter, is an excellent idea. You don't need to get tan or even pink. Be aware that sunscreen blocks vitamin D production.

### More on Vitamin $K_2$

Vitamin $K_2$ is a powerful nutrient still unknown to eaters and little understood by researchers. Vitamin $K_1$, which is essential

## THE RIGHT DOSE: VITAMINS A AND D

Someone might tell you that too much vitamin A is dangerous. Excess synthetic vitamin A has been linked to birth defects, but fears about eating foods rich in vitamin A are probably unfounded. Traditional diets contained ten times more vitamins A and D than modern diets. A 1999 study tracked more than four hundred mothers taking more than 10,000 IU of vitamin A daily—chosen because it was considered a "high" dose—during the first nine weeks of pregnancy. There were no birth defects among babies whose mothers consumed 50,000 IU.[28] However, I wouldn't take large doses of synthetic vitamin A. "While some forms of synthetic vitamin A found in supplements can be toxic at only moderately high doses, fat-soluble vitamin A naturally found in foods like cod liver oil, liver, and butterfat is safe," says Sally Fallon, founder of the Weston A. Price Foundation. The vitamin D in cod liver oil and butter protects against vitamin A toxicity. For fertility and pregnancy, the Weston A. Price Foundation recommends cod liver oil to supply 20,000 IU of vitamin A and 2,000 IU of vitamin D daily. I confess I can never remember these numbers, but I know that a daily spoonful of cod liver oil is a good dose for mothers and fathers.

for blood clotting, is more familiar. $K_1$ is found in liver and leafy greens. Its cousin vitamin $K_2$ puts calcium in the bones, where it belongs, and keeps calcium away from soft tissues like arteries, where it doesn't. Price knew that vitamin $K_2$ was important for fertility, but we're just learning how. Vitamin $K_2$ is made in large amounts from $K_1$ in the reproductive organs, which hoard vitamin $K_2$ if you don't eat enough $K_1$. We know that sperm depend on $K_2$.[29]

From fertility to bone health, vitamins A, D, and $K_2$ work together, which makes sense, because they are often found in the same foods—especially fertility foods. Vitamin $K_2$ is found in fish liver, shellfish, organ meats, and real butter. Industrial butter is not a significant source. It must be rich yellow from the carotenes in pasture. Fermented foods, such as sauerkraut, hard cheese, and natto, a traditional Japanese soy food, are outstanding vegetarian sources of $K_2$.

## More on Vitamin E

Vitamin E is the "birth vitamin." In 1924, researchers called vitamin E *tocopherol*, from the Greek, meaning "to beget or carry offspring." Price noted repeatedly that vitamin E was necessary for "reproductive efficiency" in women. It's not difficult to see why. Sperm cells need vitamin E to mature. Deficiency reduces sperm counts and quality; severe deficiency can cause sterility. Vitamin E aids sperm motility and prevents sperm from "clumping." An antioxidant, vitamin E also protects sperm from free radicals. A healthy placenta needs vitamin E, and cell division depends on it. Adelle Davis said that vitamin E prevents miscarriage when both man and woman take it for months before conception. "It markedly decreases the need for oxygen, at first meagerly supplied to the newly formed embryo," she wrote in *Let's Have Healthy Children*.

Vitamin E is found in olive oil, palm oil, avocados, almonds, wheat germ, whole grains, seeds, and leafy greens. If you take a supplement, spend money on a good one. Vitamin E supplements usually contain just alpha tocopherol, but the whole vitamin E "complex" in foods contains at least seven other agents, including beta, delta, and gamma tocopherol. According to Dr. Thomas Cowan, studies show that purified alpha tocopherol is "not nearly as effective in maintaining fertility" as real food.

## More on the B Vitamins

The whole B vitamin family is important for libido, making sex hormones, and producing eggs and sperm. Vitamin $B_{12}$ promotes sperm health and aids conception in anemic women. Vitamin $B_6$ balances estrogen and progesterone, and prevents excess prolactin. Deficiency is also associated with infertility.

The most famous baby-related B vitamin, of course, is folate. As we've mentioned, folate deficiency causes devastating defects of the brain and spinal cord before you even know you're pregnant. Every new cell needs fresh DNA, and you cannot make DNA without folate. Folate supports adequate birth weight and proper development of the heart and face. Liver, legumes, leafy greens, nuts, and chicken contain folate. Chicken liver is the most folate-rich of all livers. Synthetic supplements contain a form called folic acid. It must be converted to usable forms of folate, but this conversion is imperfect. Folic acid doesn't cross the placenta, as folate does. It's best to get folate from food, not a pill, but if you take a supplement, make sure it doesn't say "folic acid." Look for "folate" or "methylfolate."

The population in Pune, India, is largely vegetarian. They eat a lot of leafy vegetables and legumes but few animal foods. As you'd expect, pregnant women get ample folate, but 60 percent are deficient in vitamin $B_{12}$. This has a surprising effect. Women with the *highest* folate levels who were *also* deficient in vitamin $B_{12}$ had babies who were small, fat, and insulin resistant at six years. These children are much more likely to be diabetic as adults, which may explain high diabetes rates in India.[30]

This study also suggests why you probably don't need to fret about folate. In Pune, only one in seven hundred woman was deficient in folate, even though none of the women took supplements. Half of all pregnancies are unplanned. But if you eat any leaves, nuts, beans, or chicken at all, and get pregnant unexpectedly, it's very likely you had plenty of folate in the first weeks. Just a little meat, fish, milk, or eggs will cover the $B_{12}$ you need.

Folate has two other partners, betaine and choline. Both are brain nutrients. Choline is related to folate because your body can convert it to betaine, which can stand in for folate.[31] Together, choline and betaine prevent neural tube defects.[32] Choline is a major component of the neurotransmitter acetylcholine, which is essential for healthy neurons from eight weeks' gestation to three months after birth.[33] Foods rich in choline include egg yolks,

## FOODS TO AID FERTILITY AND PREVENT BIRTH DEFECTS

If you think you need a supplement, you can get all the B vitamins except $B_{12}$ from Brewer's yeast. Lewis Labs makes the one I like best.

| | |
|---|---|
| Folate | Leafy greens, liver, lentils, nuts, chicken |
| $B_6$ | Raw milk, lightly cooked liver and tuna, banana. $B_6$ is heat sensitive. |
| $B_{12}$ | Meat, fish, dairy, and eggs. $B_{12}$ is not found in plants. |
| Choline | Egg yolks, beef, wheat germ, whole grains, liver, fish |
| Betaine | Wheat germ, whole grains, spinach, beets |

beef, wheat germ, whole grains, liver, and fish. You'll find betaine in wheat germ, whole grains, spinach, and beets. Mentally, I lump folate, choline, and betaine together because their jobs are similar and they lurk in many of the same foods. You'll go crazy keeping too many lists in your head for one thing or another.

*More on Zinc*

Zinc is an all-important baby food. Mothers, fathers, and babies need it in small but steady doses in every aspect of reproductive life, from the womb to adolescence to fertility. You need zinc to make sex hormones and eggs and for a healthy thyroid. Like vitamin A, adequate zinc is essential for cell division and organ formation. You need zinc to absorb folate, which explains why spina bifida is linked to low zinc levels.

Zinc is especially critical for boys and men. Prenatal zinc deficiency prevents the male sex organs from forming properly. Men cannot make sperm without it. The prostate gland, semen, and sperm are loaded with zinc; low zinc levels in sperm are a marker of infertility. Zinc experts estimate that a man loses one milligram of zinc with every ejaculation, which means that sexually active men and teenage boys need plenty of zinc-rich foods. Dr. Cowan recommends that men with any kind of reproductive problem eat oysters once or twice a week.

After oysters, the best zinc foods are crustaceans, liver, beef, and pumpkin seeds. There is some zinc in dairy products, especially cheese. Zinc is much more effective with vitamin C, so eat plenty of raw fruit and vegetables. Another source is unrefined sea salt—not refined salt, which has been stripped of all the good sea minerals. If you don't get enough zinc, take Brewer's yeast.

## WHERE TO FIND ZINC

**The following list includes some real foods rich in zinc. There's no need to remember the numbers. I'd merely like to note the large gap between good sources (oysters) and poor ones (rice).**

|  | ZINC |
|---|---|
| Oysters | 45–70 mg per 100g |
| Liver | 7.8 |
| Brewer's yeast | 7.8 |
| Shrimp | 5.3 |
| Crab | 5.0 |
| Beef | 4.3 |
| Cheese | 4.0 |
| Peas | 0.7 |
| Carrots | 0.4 |
| Rice | 0.35 |

White spots on your fingernails are the telltale sign of zinc deficiency. In *Enhancing Fertility Naturally*, Nicky Wesson notes that certain groups, including anorexics, vegans, vegetarians, and people who eat soy instead of meat, are more likely to lack zinc. The fiber and phytic acid in soy and grains block zinc absorption. When I was (variously) too thin, vegan, and vegetarian, my finger nails had white spots. When I started to eat real food again, my nails were again a nice healthy pink. Oral contraceptives, sugar, trans fats, and the stress hormone cortisol all deplete zinc.

The RDA (recommended daily allowance) for pregnant and nursing mothers is twenty to twenty-five milligrams of zinc, but every expert in fertility foods I consulted suggests much more: fifty to eighty milligrams. In *Fertility, Cycles and Nutrition*, Marilyn Shannon writes, "Zinc is so valuable for overcoming infertility and other reproductive dysfunctions that I hesitate to limit the suggested supplement amount to twenty-five milligrams." She recommends eighty milligrams for infertility.

After reading about the nifty metal called zinc, and all the wonderful things it does for mothers, fathers, and babies, I had a new respect for the oyster. It's no accident that oysters are legendary among aphrodisiacs. But if oysters don't thrill you, don't worry. In these pages, I hope, you've found plenty of fertility foods to please your palate, perchance to conceive.

## THE SPERM TEAM

When my brother Charles and I were little, my parents read us Peter Mayle's wonderful book *"Where Did I Come From?" The Facts of Life without Any Nonsense and with Illustrations*. All the drawings are good, but the image of the Lucky Sperm always stuck with me. Swimming among countless anonymous naked sperm, he was distinguished by his shiny black top hat, jaunty bow tie, and the long-stemmed red rose he carried.

It's true. One sperm does get lucky. It penetrates the egg, driving home its genetic cargo for posterity, but the winner is more like the captain of a cycling team in the Tour de France than a lone long-distance runner. In the famously grueling French bicycle race, the team captain is aided forward by the air draft his eight teammates create ahead. It's hard work up front, bearing the brunt of oncoming wind. One by one, each exhausted rider peels off, allowing a fresh rider to lead the pack. At the very end, the leader sprints ahead to cross the finish line. He takes the prize for the team.

Sperm are similar. The vast majority of sperm will never get close to an egg, never mind fertilize it. "Most sperm produced by most men would not be able to fertilize an egg if the egg were placed directly in front of it," says the fertility specialist Dr. Bruce Rose. *Conceive* magazine says that up to 70 percent of sperm in most men are abnormal.

Hence the team effort. The silent majority of sperm propel the victor through a cervix thick with mucus and up the fallopian tubes—the equivalent of swimming one hundred miles for a man. Fully half are on the wrong track, because in a typical month, only one fallopian tube contains a mature egg. About ten hours later, just one hundred sperm, give or take a dozen, will arrive at the egg, only to encounter a jellylike layer of cells called the cumulus oophoricus. Next, a battering ram made of sperm breaks down the cumulus, allowing the guy in the top hat to inject his DNA-loaded head into the egg. Even then, the sperm that arrives first can't penetrate the egg by mere force; the eggshell is about three times thicker than a sperm head. The successful sperm carries digestive enzymes—the acrosome—to dissolve the shell. Many sperm lack the packet.

That's why the sharp decline in sperm count is so troubling. The *British Medical Journal* reported that men produce less than half the sperm their grandfathers did at the same age.[34] The average sperm count in sixty countries has fallen 42 percent since 1940, from 113 million per milliliter to 66 million. The average healthy sperm count is about 100 million per milliliter. Counts below 20 to 40 million per milliliter are considered subfertile. Semen volume and sperm quality, from head shape to swimming strength, are sinking, too.

Sperm are sensitive to heat. Sperm are born, live, and mature outside the body, in the scrotum, because they prefer a temperature cooler than 98.6 degrees Fahrenheit—89 degrees, to be precise. Too many hot saunas can damage or kill sperm. The babies of Scottish men working in a hot ceramics factory were more likely to be born preterm and have low birth weights.[35] Paternal exposure to heat causes miscarriage.[36]

Chemicals used in industrial farming imperil sperm and babies, especially boys. "Exposure of men or women to certain pesticides at sufficient doses may increase the risk for sperm abnormalities, decreased fertility, a deficit of male children, spontaneous abortion, birth defects, or fetal growth retardation," found one study.[37] Every class of pesticides is implicated. The culprit in farm chemicals is often an estrogen-like compound that disrupts male hormones.

Subfertile men have lower sperm counts if they're exposed to pesticides.[38] In farming communities of the Red River Valley of Minnesota, babies have significantly higher rates of birth defects than elsewhere. The most defects occur in the babies of men who apply pesticides.[39] The weed killer atrazine, which ends up in groundwater all over the Midwest, causes congenital stomach defects.[40] When men are exposed to pesticides, their sons are more likely to suffer from cryptorchidism, or undescended testicles.[41] Because the male fetus is more vulnerable generally, boys are literally missing from maternity wards. Researchers have spotted pollution-related boy deficits in Europe, North America, Latin America, and Asia.[42]

The chemicals to blame are not obscure poisons known only to farmers or landscaping professionals. They're for sale in the average home "improvement" store. Take a walk down that smelly gardening aisle, and you'll quickly find herbicides such as atrazine, simazine, and Roundup. Even if you don't use them on your own lawn, they're in your local groundwater and on the food you buy.

Industrial farming also threatens virility by diminishing soil health and thus the nutrients in food. In *We Want Real Food*, Graham Harvey describes how the quality of food in the United States and Europe has fallen since midcentury. Milk, beef, and eggs are missing omega-3 fats and vitamin E. Fruit and vegetables contain fewer antioxidants and less vitamin C, magnesium, calcium, zinc, iron, and copper. Synthetic fertilizer and pesticides have stripped the soil of minerals such as calcium and trace elements, such as selenium, vital to plant, animal, and human health. Sperm need these missing nutrients.

Today, fertility specialists at least nod in the direction of nutrition, if only because patients ask about it. Many recommend antioxidants to prevent damage to sperm. Dr. Marc Goldstein, professor of reproductive medicine and urology at Weill Medical College, explains, "Infertile men have a higher concentration of free radicals in their semen. Free radicals attack and destroy the membrane that surrounds sperm. Antioxidants fight these bad effects. Vitamins are natural antioxidants."

Goldstein prescribes the antioxidant $CoQ_{10}$, folic acid, vitamins C and E, selenium, and zinc to subfertile men. He also recommends lycopene, an antioxidant found in high concentrations in semen and L-carnitine, an amino acid sperm use for energy. There is lycopene in tomatoes and L-carnitine in meat.

All these nutrients are pro-baby. Vitamin E improves sperm motility and form, and vitamin C prevents oxidation of E. You need folate to make RNA, DNA, and new cells. In one study, zinc and folic acid nearly doubled sperm counts in subfertile men, and raised it in fertile men, too.[43] The doses in this trial were large: five thousand micrograms of folic acid and sixty-six grams of zinc. Low folate levels predict problems with sperm chromosomes in men of all ages. Men consuming the most folate— from 700 to nearly 1,200 micrograms daily—have 20 to 30 percent fewer sperm abnormalities.[44] You cannot make testosterone without the antioxidant selenium, which is found in high concentrations in semen. The protein that forms the midsection of the sperm tail is made from selenium; without this nutrient, sperm are sterile. Selenium also renders sperm-killing methylmercury inactive.

Men may wish to avoid estrogen-rich soy. The Israeli Health Ministry warns men to "exercise caution" regarding soy

## FERTILITY NUTRIENTS FOR MEN

| | BENEFITS | FOODS | PILLS, ETC. |
|---|---|---|---|
| Antioxidants | Healthy sperm | Fruit, vegetables, nuts, spices, tea | Raw juice, CoQ$_{10}$ |
| Vitamin C | Healthy sperm | Fruit, vegetables | Vitamin C |
| Vitamin E | Healthy sperm | Olive oil, nuts | Vitamin E |
| Folate | DNA and RNA | Liver, leaves, lentils, nuts, chicken | Brewer's yeast, methylfolate |
| Iron | Protein, DNA | Red meat, liver | Brewer's yeast, Floradix |
| Omega-3 fats | Healthy sperm | Fish, roe | Fish oil |
| Selenium | Testosterone | Brazil nuts, beef, tuna | Brewer's yeast |
| Zinc | Healthy sperm | Oysters, beef, shrimp | Brewer's yeast |

consumption because of its effects on virility. Again the trouble is plant estrogens. Excess estrogen in the womb causes abnormal sexual development and low sperm counts in boys and men. Eating soy reduces testosterone and raises estrogen in men.[45] In one study of subfertile men, those eating the most soy had about forty-one million fewer sperm per milliliter than men who consumed none.[46] The damaging dose was small. Over the three months before giving a semen sample, soy eaters said they ate about one half serving of soy foods daily, the equivalent of half a tofu patty. Strict vegetarian diets are linked to male infertility due to zinc deficiency. (Recall that phytic acid in soy blocks zinc.) If you must eat soy, choose traditional foods, not soy protein.

Last but not least, excess weight can interfere with fatherhood. Extra fat lowers testosterone, raises estrogen, and lowers the number of strong swimmers in semen. Among farmers, fertility declines as body mass index rises.[47] In 2011, Reproductive BioMedicine online published a study linking a body mass index (BMI) of thirty or more to lower sperm counts and abnormal sperm.

For men, the pro-baby plan is pretty simple. If you'd like to be a father, keep the sperm team in fighting shape by eating plenty of real food rich in antioxidants. Don't use chemicals on your lawn. Buy ecological foods when you can. Stay trim.

## A POPULATION OF ONE

In my single days, one pleasure in my life was car trips with my parents. In February of 2006, we set out from New York City to State College, Pennsylvania, for the annual conference of the Pennsylvania Association for Sustainable Agriculture, one of the best gatherings for farmers and ranchers who raise real food. The weather was bad, as it always seems to be in the Pennsylvania hills that time of year, so we drove gently, but we had reasons to be cheerful. Winter is the off-season for vegetable farmers. We knew we'd see many farming friends, and the seminars—on organic orchards or grazing or cheese making—are always enlightening.

Plus, the food is good. Some time ago, PASA and other local-food groups started to put the catering budget where it belongs: in the pockets of local farmers. There's no point in talking real food when you're eating corn syrup. Nowadays there's always plenty of real food at these gatherings, from raw milk cheese to grass-fed beef. You've never eaten so well in a big hotel.

Dennis Wolff, the secretary of the Pennsylvania Department of Agriculture, spoke at the final banquet. He talked as politicians will, playing to the crowd and crowing about his accomplishments. Allow me to paraphrase the memorable bits. *There are more organic farmers in Pennsylvania than last year.* Polite applause. *There are more women farming than ever before.* Murmurs of approval. *Last year,* said the secretary, *we licensed a record number of dairies to sell raw milk in Pennsylvania.* Thunderous applause. You see why we enjoy this meeting.

I'd never heard of the keynote speaker, but the minute I saw her name I knew I'd better get to know her work. Sandra Steingraber is a biologist, cancer survivor, poet, and expert in a particular ecology: that of the womb. She began her talk to an audience of hundreds by calling all the nursing mothers and babies who might've slunk out, presumably for fear of making too much noise, back into the lecture hall. We cheered. Then Steingraber moved swiftly on to a poetic and scientifically precise account of what was going on inside me.

I didn't know it, of course, but by lunchtime on Friday, February 3, I was One Day Pregnant—or about to be. It is not a precise business. Eggs are transient creatures, dead after twelve or (at most) twenty-four hours, but sperm may live inside a woman for five days, so it's difficult to pinpoint the moment of conception from whatever you might've written in your diary, still less from the first day you realize your period is late. That's why midwives and obstetricians count the forty weeks of human gestation from the first day of your last period, not the day *you* happen to think your egg got the Kiss.

The process embryologists call fertilization is not a single moment anyway; it takes twelve to twenty-four hours. Ten hours go by while the sperm travels up the fallopian tubes. The egg is hardly passive, however. One of the largest cells in the body, the egg uses its own means to travel *down* the fallopian tubes. An egg without a healthy outer coating doesn't move at all. Or, just as likely, the whole crowd of sperm may get there first, only to wait for a mature egg to be released, bubblelike, from the ovarian wands, to be drawn into the waiting fallopian tubes by fluttering cilia.

However the two main characters meet, there is some pushing and shoving before the successful sperm delivers its twenty-three chromosomes, with what I imagine to be a sort of *whoosh* as the sperm head is irretrievably sucked into the egg. In the next instant, there's a kind of zipping sound (or so I hear it) as the egg seals over, blocking all latecomers forever. When it's done, the sperm and egg are a zygote, a single-celled creature.

As Steingraber was speaking, a tiny new life was gearing up in my belly. Within a day of conception, the zygote begins to cleave: one cell becomes two, two become four, four become eight. At first, the pace is calm; each division comes some twenty hours after the last. About four days after conception, the zygote comprises about sixteen cells; it's now called a morula, from the Latin for mulberry. Still dividing—only now, thanks to the wonders of geometric progression, with dramatic results—the tiny ball of cells wends its way to the uterus to make a home on day five or six or maybe seven. Now it's called a blastocyst, and pregnancy is really under way.

A simple and inexpensive pregnancy test will allow you to confirm this as soon as the embryo sinks into the uterus by detecting a hormone called human chorionic gonadotropin (HCG), found helpfully enough right in your pee within days of missing your period. Even though the whole of this new living thing is merely 0.1 to 0.2 millimeters across, it already contains an unimaginably tiny placenta, which begins to release HCG when the blastocyst gets comfortable in the rich, soft endometrium. HCG has a simple job: It tells your body to keep pumping progesterone ("pro-gestation") and to call off your period. This time, the blood stays inside.

In *Having Faith: An Ecologist's Journey into Motherhood*, Steingraber describes the aftermath of conception.

> One week after the egg's successful affair with the sperm, the whole unit sinks into the endometrial marsh in a process called implantation. The fused cells push long, amoeba-like fingers deep into the uterine lining while secreting digestive enzymes that facilitate its burial. In response, the tips of the spiral arteries break open and spurt like geysers. Thus, life begins in a pool of blood.

The new life the egg and sperm created only days ago—a microscopic, hidden life you don't even know about yet—now devours the inside layer of your uterus to burrow beneath it, the better to secure a safe perch and steady supply of blood for oxygen and nutrients.

Pregnant women may be accused of navel-gazing, but you'd need the imagination of a lentil not to feel a shred of wonder at the torrent of microscopic activity roiling away just beneath your very own navel—the same navel that was your lifeline to your own mother, decades ago.

I listened transfixed, taking the occasional note, as Steingraber's story turned from wondrous to something darker. On finding herself pregnant, this ecologist suddenly became an expert in the smallest environment: the womb. "I had become a habitat," I heard her say, "with a population of one."

Conditions in this tiny environment—a healthy womb is the size of a large fig or a small pear when the baby settles there—directly affect the development of the baby's organs, bones, eyes, brain, and more. Unfortunately, the womb is polluted beyond dispute. Some effects are far-reaching and unexpected. For example, poor mineral levels in a child's first molars are the best measure of prenatal dioxin exposure.[48]

Steingraber told a hall full of farmers a few things about what farm chemicals do to mothers, fathers, babies, and kids. Pesticides lower sperm counts, interfere with the implantation of the embryo, and cause preterm labor. Farmers and farmers' kids have higher rates of birth defects and pediatric and adult cancers.

Most, if not all, of the hundreds of farmers listening that day favored ecological methods, but I reckon we had all eaten lots of food with pesticide residues and we all knew plenty about pesticide drift from other farms. I thought guiltily of the chemicals we used to use when I was little: the Roundup we sprayed on Johnson grass, atrazine and simazine on sweet corn. The half-life of atrazine in the soil is two weeks to one hundred days. Simazine stays in the soil for two to seven months. We stopped growing sweet corn when we gave up chemicals. Hand-weeding and hoeing corn was not a sensible use of precious labor.

To hear the chemical companies tell it, under a certain limit these poisons have no effect. The dose has to be extreme, exposure excessive. But that is the old theory of toxicity: The dose makes the poison. Now we know that even a small dose is not necessarily a safe one. With unborn babies in particular, timing makes the poison. Windows of development—organ synthesis, brain growth, sexual maturity—are so exquisitely sensitive that exposure to toxins can have devastating effects.

The tragedy of thalidomide, a drug many pregnant women took in the 1950s to ease nausea, illustrates just how sensitive. The critical window for thalidomide damage turned out to be thirty-five to fifty days after a woman's last period. Precisely when the mother took the drug predicted what particular disaster befell her baby. "Embryos develop from the head down and the center out," writes Steingraber. "Thus, pills taken between days 35 to 37 resulted in babies with no ears, whereas pills taken between days 39 to 41 resulted in no arms. Days 41 to 43, no uterus. Days 45 to 47, no leg bones. Days 47 to 49, deformed thumbs." For the delicate embryo, the stakes are unimaginably high.

The fetal brain, too, is uniquely vulnerable, more so than the child or adult brain. Your body has many layers of protection from poisons and pathogens. The skin forms an initial barrier. Inside the body, protective bacteria coat the intestines, the liver detoxifies, the kidney eliminates. Another filter is called the blood-brain barrier. If a toxin contaminates the blood, this barrier prevents it from passing from the blood to the brain, where it may do serious damage. Not in the fetus. There is no blood-brain barrier until the sixth month of pregnancy.

You may recall that you can't absorb fat-soluble vitamins, such as vitamin D, without fat. But there is a flip side to fat. Fat attracts and accumulates fat-soluble poisons just as readily as nutrients. This has unhappy implications for the baby's brain. Until the eighth or ninth month, the fetus is lean. Its main activity is building organs, bone, muscle, and brain. The final weeks are for packing on body fat, the better to stay warm and survive possible interruptions in the food supply outside the womb. But the brain is the house that fat built: It is 50 to 60 percent fat by weight. Fat-soluble toxins cannot settle in a lean fetus, so they lodge in the baby's brain.

When I found out I was pregnant, just eleven days after hearing these harrowing facts, I thought I would never eat pesticide-ridden industrial foods again. My mother bought *Having Faith* at the conference, dug in, and implored me to read it. Dad took the other view: "A book about the effects of environmental toxins on fetal health is the last thing a pregnant woman needs."

For the next nine months, I tried—as I usually try—to avoid industrial foods, chemicals, vapors, smoke, pesticides, and any kind of junk you can put in or on your body. I also avoided Steingraber's book. I could have worried myself silly about the toxins in my fat, but they weren't going anywhere fast. The baby would be here, in one state or another, before the pollutants broke down. It seemed sensible to concentrate on things I could control, namely the foods the baby needed right now. It also seemed sensible to worry less. I left *Having Faith* on the shelf.

And that is what I recommend. Do read this superb book, preferably well before you get pregnant. If you're already pregnant and (like me) you're sensitive about these things, you might wait until after your baby is born. Or ask the baby's father to read it. It cannot fail to rouse him to his natural and primitive state, fierce about defending his mate and babies from perils of all kinds. I'm quite serious. Pregnant women, mothers, and babies need protectors and advocates, at home and away from it.

Meanwhile, consider cleaning up at home. An unborn baby occupies a series of layered habitats, like a set of Russian nesting dolls. Her immediate home is your womb. She floats in amniotic fluid you make. She drinks it, pees in it, drinks it again. She gets food and oxygen from your blood. What you eat and drink, she eats and drinks. Perhaps there is lead in the water, or trans fat in the "buttery" spread, or pesticide residue on the apples. Your home is the baby's next habitat. Does it smell like the cleanser aisle at the supermarket? Maybe you're ready to buy organic cotton, ban chlorine at home, or hand wash woolens with lanolin, instead of taking them to the dry cleaner.

Cleaning up at the next level—the neighborhood, nation, world—is a larger civic project. I'm always a little hopeful. After all, unbiased research and political action did, eventually, rid the world of things known to harm babies, such as lead paint, DDT, and thalidomide—all banned. Now we can turn our attention to threats such as cell phone radiation and methylmercury, which comes from trash burning and ends up in fish.

## CHAPTER 3

# Forty Weeks

**MOTHER AND BABY IN THE FIRST TRIMESTER**

You're a few weeks pregnant. It's exciting. For a while, maybe months, it's probably a family secret. Many women feel wonderful. Other women feel not-so-wonderful. It's common to feel breathless, constipated, nauseated, and sleepy—as if drugged. All this is normal. These symptoms represent a host of interior changes, including surging hormones and expanding fluids. Lots of action, all of it inside. Perhaps your breasts are a bit plumper. (That can be fun.) But there's nothing else to see.

The embryo, growing furiously, is still the size of a dime, a kidney bean, a marble . . . you can learn all this from week-by-week pregnancy calendars, but I don't care for them. They mostly want to sell you something. They make too much fuss over little changes. They keep your head in the twigs, never mind the forest. Pregnancy is an indivisible, organic condition. Weeks don't matter. Even the trimesters—twelve to fourteen weeks each—don't correspond to embryological milestones.

It may be that all you want to do is lie down. When you're in that kind of mood, reading book after book about what you need to eat and what can go wrong seems . . . counterproductive. I also think shopping for baby items is premature, but that's a matter of preference. Ahead of you are years of baby-related activities. If you can, divert your mind with nonbaby matters. When you and your brain wake up, perhaps you'll be eager to consume lots of pregnancy-related stuff.

Prenatal nutrition in particular can be overwhelming. So much to eat, so many reasons why. I found it all too much, and from what I hear, I'm not alone. There is no need to feel deluged by the information. When I couldn't face any more advice about what to eat, I devised my own scheme. Here's a quick sketch of how I think about eating for two.

You have about forty weeks to build a baby. Since we're all steeped in the language of trimesters, let's assume it happens in three acts. Your baby's parts—her tiny liver, lungs, toes—are made of micronutrients called vitamins, so you hardly need to eat anything extra in the first trimester. Just eat well. If that's difficult, take well-chosen supplements. Your baby's structure—his bone and muscle—are made of calcium and protein, so have plenty of both in the second trimester. Your baby's brain is made of fish, so it's important to eat plenty of seafood at the end. Of course you'll want to eat well all the while, and this cartoon of fetal development is certainly oversimplified. It may seem silly at first, but there is logic in it, and it worked for me.

## KNOCKED OUT LOADED

When I got pregnant, I had just finished writing *Real Food*. I was thoroughly immersed in basic nutrition, and I had a fair idea of what pregnant women, nursing mothers, and babies needed. Nevertheless, overconfidence isn't a good trait, so I thought I'd check out what the experts had to say about what to eat when you're expecting.

They should call these books "what to make yourself eat when you're expecting." It's not enough to eat well. You will be "eating for two." You should also expect weird cravings for some foods and powerful aversions to others. The baby's father will have to make junk food runs at midnight when you demand wacky flavor combinations.

This was not my experience.

I was alarmed by the nutritional advice for pregnancy. Not because the experts got things wrong—although here and there, I did disagree—but because the amount of food they told me to eat was two or three times greater than I could ever manage. I'm not talking about the three to five hundred "extra" calories they recommend you eat, which is not even necessary for the first twelve weeks—unless you're too thin or ravenous, in which case, by all means, eat. Three hundred calories isn't much; it amounts to a yogurt and a handful of nuts. My appetite didn't change an iota until about fourteen weeks. Then I was occasionally hungry for more, but for just a little more.

No. I'm only talking about adding up all the foods said to be essential. In one book, this was the daily menu:

* 4 servings of protein
* 2 servings of vitamin C foods
* 4 servings of calcium foods
* 3 servings of green and yellow foods
* 1–2 servings of other vegetables
* 6 or more servings of complex carbohydrates
* 2 servings of "high-fat" foods
* Some iron-rich foods

It's all healthy food and reasonable, but I was not even interested in eating for one, much less two. (The second time, with twins, was another story.) Feeling not too hungry is a typical symptom of early pregnancy. An early sign of pregnancy is elevated progesterone. This hormone builds up the uterine lining, slightly suppresses immune response so as not to reject the baby as a foreign invader, reduces uterine contractions, and suppresses lactation. Progesterone also slows down the digestive tract to make sure your body gets every nutrient from the food you eat. The hormone relaxin, whose main job is to relax your joints, thus permitting your pelvis to widen gently, also alters the membranes of your intestine to slow digestion and grab every nutrient you consume. Clever nature!

Ah, but another way to describe this is constipation. It's hard to feel hungry for all that food when you don't seem to be finished with the food you just ate. In the early weeks, I often had a lead stomach. I knew that meat was important for building new blood—my diary says, "Eat more beef!"—but even one serving was beyond my appetite, never mind four. Eating six portions of bread and rice was out of the question. All I wanted was fruit, salads, broth, and lots of water. Constipation may persist, so find a strategy that works for you.

Progesterone is also a sedative. You may sleep long and soundly and feel drowsy by day. This bland description doesn't do justice to reality. I kept thinking of the Bob Dylan song "Under Your Spell" as I dragged my leaden body around: "I was knocked out loaded in the naked night." My tiny, invisible cargo flattened me. I slept nine hours a night, then ten, and then eleven—plus one- and two-hour naps, and I had never been a napper. Morning would come, and I couldn't budge. By day I often found it necessary to lie down. I did a lot of business flat on my back on the phone. I began to wonder whether I'd be able to make a living in my waning productive hours. When I woke up from these long, druglike slumbers, I wasn't at all hungry.

As for the two permitted servings of "high-fat" foods, these were some of the few foods I *did* make room for. I was confident that eating grass-fed butter, coconut oil, and other good fats more than the twice daily recommended was good, but fats are filling, and they left me little room for other foods.

On the other hand, pregnancy books were, in some ways, blasé about nutrition. "Eat whatever you can, even if that means nothing but ginger ale, Popsicles, and hard candy," said one dietician. "Your digestive system is very effective at capturing calories." At capturing calories, sure. What about nutrients? Where the other advice about what to eat was too precise, bossy, and hard to follow, this was the nutritional equivalent of throwing in the towel. Those three things are pure sugar, and sugar isn't good for mother or baby. Probably better to eat nothing. Your teeny-tiny baby doesn't need any calories yet, and eventually, you'll be hungry for some small amount of real food, like a cashew—which happens to contain folate, I might add.

For views closer to my own, I looked up the prenatal diet recommended by the Weston A. Price Foundation. There were no surprises, nutritionally speaking, but again the daily dose seemed gargantuan.

* 1 T cod liver oil daily for vitamins A and D
* 2 T coconut oil daily for lauric acid
* 4 T butter daily for saturated fats and vitamin A
* 2 glasses raw milk daily for calcium
* 2 or more eggs plus extra egg yolks daily for protein and vitamin A
* Beef or lamb daily for B vitamins, iron, and protein
* Oily fish or lard daily for vitamin D
* Liver once or twice a week for B vitamins, iron, and protein
* Fish and roe two to four times a week for omega-3 fats, iodine, and protein

I found this list so intimidating, I didn't even write down the grains, fruit, and vegetables, which I could easily remember, just the fats and protein. I typed it up just as you see it here, and put it on my fridge and in my wallet. Then I tried the diet.

Impossible. I couldn't even manage it for one full day. I had all the foods in fridge and pantry, but this menu gave me problems. Again, it was too much. Also, I didn't like beef and lamb enough to eat them daily, though I do now. Fish and chicken, maybe. Beef twice a week—I could do that. I found myself whining about eating lamb. Finally, I could not, no matter how I tried, find a way to use lard daily. And I'm unusual in that I buy, cook with, enjoy—and approve of—pig fat.

Next I turned to Adelle Davis, author of no-nonsense best-sellers on nutrition in the 1950s and 1960s. Some of her views are dated. Now we know that powdered milk isn't good for you, and that when she says "vegetable oil," you should think of cold-pressed olive oil, not corn oil. Yet of all the authors on the pop nutrition shelf, Davis still has superior advice. I thumbed a dog-eared copy of her 1951 classic, *Let's Have Healthy Children*. For Davis, the prenatal menu is simple, and I liked the way she arranged it.

**BREAKFAST**
* Fruit
* Brewer's yeast in milk or juice
* Whole grain toast
* If hungry: eggs, yogurt, wheat germ, whole grain cereal, liver, meat, poultry, or fish

**LUNCH**
* Brewer's yeast in milk or juice
* Yogurt with fruit
* Meat, poultry, fish, eggs, cottage cheese, or peanut butter
* Salad or vegetables with olive oil or mayonnaise

**DINNER**
* Meat, poultry, fish, or soup made with milk or meat
* Cooked vegetables, especially leafy greens
* Salad with dressing
* Milk, yogurt, or buttermilk
* If hungry: fruit

This eating plan seemed doable. Davis emphasized the elements you needed to build a baby: vitamins, protein, calcium. She suggested you fill in with the rest, according to taste and hunger: fruit, brown rice, whole wheat toast, chocolate. (True, she never mentioned chocolate, but women who eat chocolate daily when they're pregnant have babies who smile more.)[1]

Still, a few items raised eyebrows. Davis recommends a daily "pep-up" shake containing two cups milk, powdered milk, vegetable oil, a half cup of yeast, a half cup of fruit, two raw eggs, vanilla, and—yes—half an eggshell. After blending these ingredients, you're to add another two quarts of milk and sip all day. She made a big point of eating liver, too.

By this stage, I was overfed with nutrition information, but I was determined to be a Good Eater and willing to follow instructions. For a few weeks, I dutifully ate liver twice a week. To make room for all the beef, chicken, fish, eggs, cheese, milk, and butter, I reluctantly cut way back on dark chocolate (to a couple of squares), fresh fruit (from five or six pieces down to two or three), and homemade ice cream, now with a mere smidgen of honey or maple syrup.

Still, I wasn't happy. Meals were not a pleasure. Thinking about nutrition all the time was nerve-wracking and time-consuming. I worried about neglecting some vital nutrient. But mostly, it was too much food.

Something didn't seem right. Could it really be necessary to eat like this? We've been having babies much longer than we've understood iron or vitamin D. For my own peace of mind, it was time for me to think about baby food another way. That's how I came up with my simplified view of the baby's nutritional needs in the three trimesters: first vitamins, then protein and calcium, and finally, fish. At last confident my baby had what it needed, I could relax. A relaxed mother is just what a baby needs.

Your baby's tiny parts—organs, limbs—are made of vitamins, or rather cannot form without them. By three or four weeks, the spinal cord has formed, thanks to B vitamins. At six weeks, the baby has buds for arms and legs and the beginnings of every major organ, from heart to lungs. Organs and limbs depend on vitamin A.[2] Research at the Salk Institute for Biological Studies finds that vitamin A is also responsible for the fact that the body is symmetrical on the outside (two arms, two legs) and

## A QUICK LOOK AT FORTY WEEKS

|  | THE BABY NEEDS | BEST FOODS | PILLS, ETC. |
| --- | --- | --- | --- |
| All Along | B vitamins | Meat, poultry, lentils, whole grains | Brewer's yeast |
|  | Vitamin C | Fruit, vegetables | Vitamin C |
|  | Vitamin E | Olive oil, nuts | Vitamin E |
| Act 1 | Vitamins A and D; folate | Butter, eggs, pork, sea-food; liver, leafy greens | Cod liver oil; methylfolate |
| Act 2 | Calcium and protein | Meat, fish, poultry, milk, cheese, eggs | Whey |
| Act 3 | Omega-3 fats | Fish | Fish oil |

asymmetrical on the inside (one off-center heart). Vitamin C builds tissues, including a strong uterus. Vitamins A and E are required for DNA and RNA synthesis. Every new cell needs newly minted DNA and RNA.

If you get the *micro*nutrients you need in these early weeks, it won't matter much if you can't or don't care to eat large amounts of the *macro*nutrients (protein, fat, carbohydrates). Eating a little real food is good enough. Even my slightest meals—salad with olive oil, or zucchini with butter, followed by fruit or milk—provided plenty of folate and fat-soluble vitamins. But if you're fretful, as I was—no doubt needlessly, given how well fed I was before I conceived—this is the perfect time for supplements.

As long as I was taking cod liver oil, I realized, I didn't need to eat liver twice a week for vitamins A and D. Taking cod liver oil in the first trimester is associated with higher birth weight, even after adjusting for variables such as length of gestation.[3] As long as I had a little grass-fed butter oil, which contains vitamins A and $K_2$, I didn't need to worry about whether there was enough butter on my eggs. I could probably skip the extra lard altogether. (Hurrah!) When I took fish oil, I didn't worry if I wasn't hungry for salmon. Brewer's yeast could stand in—if only temporarily—for some of the B vitamins, zinc, and iron in red meat.

When you do eat, make it real food. Any junk you eat is a waste of calories because it gives you and the baby no nutrients and depletes you of others. White flour is useless and sugar downright harmful. (Both use up B vitamins.) Don't be a prig about junk food, but keep it to a minimum. Good ice cream and dark chocolate are excellent treats.

Please don't fall for pregnancy-related junk food. I saw an "all-natural" pregnancy snack "recommended by ob-gyns" described as "nutritious, bite-sized chews." The first three ingredients in the chocolate flavor were corn syrup, sugar, and sweetened condensed milk. When I buy chocolate, I like to see chocolate as the first ingredient, not the fourth. The pregnancy gimmick was DHA made from algae.

Nor can I recommend "improved" foods. "Enriched" means adding back the nutrients lost during refining. "Fortified" means adding more nutrients. I suppose we can be grateful that these foods contain some of the nutrients lost since industrial farming and industrial food took over, but they're not ideal. Often, nutrients in these engineered foods don't come in the ideal combination. The calcium added to orange juice, for example, cannot be absorbed without fat. Moreover, these foods generally contain the cheapest form of the added nutrient. The best supplements, such as cod liver oil and Brewer's yeast, come from real food.

There is too much advice about how much to eat and when. Said one book, "Ordinarily it's okay to have tea and toast for a day or two when you have the flu, but that's *not* okay when you're pregnant." Oh, really? Terrifying, the idea of "starving" your baby because you're too selfish to eat, but I don't buy it. In the first trimester, the fetus doesn't need extra calories. It can thrive on your stores even if you're eating poorly or not at all. If you feel better eating small, frequent meals, by all means, do. But snacks are not mandatory, either. Later, you may be ravenous—or not. Follow your appetite. If you're not hungry, you may even lose a pound or two at first. That's OK.

Slow down and take the long view. You have forty weeks to eat well. It's better not to think about daily consumption of any nutrient or any food. The fabulous, abundant banquet of good foods in pregnancy books, including this one, is just a notion, a list of options to encourage you. No matter what they say, you simply do not need to eat all these foods every day, and you'll be miserable if you try. Over time, diversity at dinner is good, but don't make a fetish of it. At a given meal, you'll eat one or two foods, not twelve—perhaps a bowl of tomato soup, egg salad on toast, steak and salad. You might even eat the same food at the next meal. That's normal and healthy, even when you're pregnant.

## MORE BLOOD

One Saturday in March, Rob bought us tickets to see the Shirelles at a small, unhip venue in Chelsea. We're suckers for Motown and all its relations, and were amazed that this 1960s act, however wrinkly, was still going. The four-girl group from Passaic, New Jersey, got together in 1958 and had a string of hits, including "Baby, It's You" and the one Carole King made famous, "Will You Love Me Tomorrow?"

The lobby was packed. "Standing room only," barked the bouncer. "People with tickets, get in line." We made our way to the end of a long line. I was seven weeks pregnant, and Rob's protective instincts flared. He went looking for the head bouncer, whose efficiency was matched only by a lack of visible emotion. "My girlfriend is pregnant, and she needs to sit down," he said firmly. "Can you make that happen?"

The bouncer was typical: lean, muscular, square of jaw, and practiced at deflecting incoming nonsense of all kinds. She shot Rob a skeptical look and told him to cool his heels. I stood in line while a determined Rob set off. As VIPs made it past the ropes, my hopes sank. I got ready to slip off my heels and lean delicately against the bar, like a wilting orchid. Twenty minutes later, Rob came looking for me, having prevailed over other ordinary citizens who arrived before we did.

We sat down, thighs pressed against each other's and everyone else's, and enjoyed an attenuated version of the once bouncy Shirelles, minus the famous Shirley. I had half a glass of wine diluted with sparkling water, my first drink since finding out I was pregnant. We were jolly. As we left, the bouncer looked me over, resting her narrow eyes on my flat belly. "You the one who's pregnant?" I nodded, attempting to convey modesty and gratitude, without looking pathetic.

"Yeah," she said. "Sometimes that works."

In fact we weren't crying wolf. Within days of getting pregnant, I was lightheaded. When I stood up quickly, I nearly fell over. When I crossed the street quickly to make the light, I was huffing and puffing. Only days before, I was plenty fit, and now I was dizzy and panting. Disconcerting. But I didn't find the answer in any conventional pregnancy book.

Turns out, I had "orthostatic hypotension," the technical term for temporary low blood pressure on standing upright. This is quite normal. Pregnancy hormones relax blood vessels to prepare for the large increase in blood volume. But the extra hemoglobin, water, salt, and other elements of blood haven't arrived yet, so you suffer from "underfill." When you stand up, blood doesn't reach your head immediately. Moreover, large amounts of blood and oxygen are being diverted to the placenta.

When it comes to blood and oxygen, the baby is first in line. The huffing, meanwhile, was caused by extra progesterone, which makes you breathe more, to get more oxygen to the baby and clear carbon dioxide faster.

Maybe reading all this makes you want to lie down. Oddly enough, the best medicine for these symptoms is exercise—when you're ready. We used to think that moderate exercise in pregnancy was merely safe, and that's what the books mostly say. But a dogged researcher named Dr. James Clapp discovered that the effects of exercise duplicate and—curiously—complement the changes of pregnancy. A pregnant woman has expanded blood volume, more blood flow to the skin, larger heart chambers, greater blood volume per heartbeat, and faster transfer of oxygen to tissues. So does an athlete. These overlapping effects are good for mother and baby. They hasten the changes the baby is calling for.

It's best if you're fit before you conceive. Blood volume and red blood cells are 10 to 15 percent greater in fit pregnant women than in sedentary ones. Put another way, the fit woman adjusts to pregnancy faster. But if you're already pregnant and out of shape, be encouraged. Women who start exercise midway through pregnancy get some benefits, just not quite as many as those who are active all along.

What are those benefits? Active women gain less weight and less fat. They have easier, shorter, and less complicated labor. They're more likely to go into labor naturally, and less likely to need medicine for pain, get an episiotomy, have a forceps delivery, or need a cesarean section. These labor-related benefits disappear if you stop exercising midway through pregnancy. After birth, women who exercise lose weight more easily.

Babies benefit from exercise, too. The placenta grows faster, which means more blood, oxygen, and nutrients get to the baby. Training reduces prematurity and low birth weight, probably because it improves glucose delivery to the baby. At birth, one year, and five years, the babies of women who exercise are as healthy as the babies of sedentary ones by several measures. The active babies are also slightly leaner at birth. Leanness—in contrast to low birth weight—may protect against obesity, diabetes, and heart disease.

All these benefits come from regular, sustained, weight-bearing, and aerobic exercise. Walking, running, swimming, dancing, cycling, rowing, or hiking will do it. If you're nervous, as I was, about all that bouncing around when you run, it's nice to know that miscarriage is not more common when mothers exercise. According to Clapp, yoga has never been studied properly. But the experience of countless mothers indicates that prenatal yoga is safe and probably beneficial.

How much you exercise is up to you. Athletes at all levels (casual, moderate, and competitive) get these benefits. Do enough to feel an effect—some work and some reward—but never to the point of fatigue. *Do not exercise when in pain, injured, or bleeding.* Clapp suggests adding at least one hour of rest, either sleeping or merely lying down, for each hour of exercise. This is sterling advice. Finally, don't follow a rigid program. Pregnancy is a variable state. It pays to make frequent adjustments.

From zero to forty weeks, I exercised four to six days a week. I walked for hours, went jogging for thirty minutes or more, and practiced yoga for an hour or more. At thirty-nine weeks, I was still running—just more gently than before, and usually indoors on the treadmill, instead of along the river. After every bout of exercise—even walking—I rested a lot.

One day, I walked to TriBeCa to take a class from the master teacher who had trained my own instructor, the wonderful Beth, in prenatal yoga. She was marvelous, as Beth had promised, but I was annoyed. It was a long walk, the class cost thirty dollars, and I wasn't that good at any of it, especially one wall maneuver with a loud, yogic breath. After class, I wandered through the fancy shop, feeling unfashionable and irritable, but too grumpy to go home. I was alienated and doubtful about the whole prenatal industry.

A woman from our class caught my eye, and we started to talk. Molly was a professional dancer and fifty times fitter than I was, but we found common ground. Like me, she had fretted about staying in shape during pregnancy and was glad to learn it was not only safe but smart. She was also the only woman I'd met who shared my hopes for a natural birth, so I found myself unusually chatty. We talked awhile, nodding a lot. Our due dates were close, and we parted promising to e-mail with baby news.

Suddenly, the little waiting room filled with strollers. It was time for mother and baby yoga. I stared through the curtain at the wriggling, mewling larvae, struck at last by baby lust. Although I'd wanted my own baby forever, I'd never really looked at babies. Faith restored, I marched home humming. In nine months, it was the best thirty dollars I spent.

## A GLASS OF WINE?

These are the early days, the days of tiny parts. We cannot fail to mention the most famous teratogen—something that causes birth defects—that can also be called a traditional food. That is ethanol, otherwise known as wine, beer, or spirits. In the United States, the surgeon general warns pregnant women not to drink any alcohol whatsoever. Every bottle of alcohol bears this stern label: WOMEN SHOULD NOT DRINK ALCOHOLIC BEVERAGES DURING PREGNANCY BECAUSE OF THE RISK OF BIRTH DEFECTS.

Limitations on maternal drinking are as old as booze. In Judges, God appears to Manoah's wife. "You are sterile and childless," he says. "But you are going to conceive and have a son. Now see to it that you drink no wine or other fermented drink." (She does have a boy and calls him Samson.) In the eighteenth and nineteenth centuries, British public health advocates deplored boozing in pregnant women. In 1834, the House of Commons declared—in a paper called "Effects of Drunkenness on the Nation"—that babies of drunks tend to be "starved, shriveled, and imperfect in form."[4]

Alcohol is relatively recent, and its abundance quite recent, which together suggest that rare to moderate consumption is traditional. Hunter-gatherers had little chance to get drunk. In the Stone Age, exposure to alcohol, probably from fermented honey or fruits, would have been rare at most.[5] We can assume these drinks were neither strong nor readily available.

Alcohol became common when people began to farm and grow grains, fruit, and other starches worth fermenting. The rise of farming, plus the invention of ceramics to store drinks, led quickly to widespread alcohol use. Humans brewed barley beer in the Near East 7,500 years ago; 3,000 years later, 40 percent of the grain crop in ancient Sumer was used to make beer. The Egyptians appear to have made the first wine from grapes. Later, the Babylonians used dates and the Chinese, rice.

Drinking is here to stay. Its fans are many. I consider alcohol one of the top four food-drugs, along with cayenne, chocolate, and caffeine. A drug it is, without question. However, the evidence that prenatal drinking is bad for babies is not entirely satisfactory. The only proper studies have been conducted on heavy drinkers. For these studies, we are grateful. It's clear that heavy and chronic drinking—and probably binge boozing—during pregnancy poisons the tiny baby's entire body. Symptoms of the devastating condition called fetal alcohol syndrome include small head and brain, facial abnormalities, organ defects, and neurodevelopmental abnormalities including impaired fine motor skills, abnormal walking, hearing loss, and poor eye-hand coordination.

The problem is dose and timing. How much alcohol is too much? How rapidly does a particular woman metabolize alcohol? What if she's eating, too? Because it's not ethical to conduct randomized, controlled studies on pregnant women, little research has answered these questions. The U.S. government, conservatively, makes no distinction between light, moderate, and heavy drinking. In fact, clinically speaking, there is no definition of "light" or "moderate" drinking in pregnancy.

The blanket prohibition against drinking, combined with anecdotal and firsthand evidence from many generations of women, has a noticeable result. Many women, and even some obstetricians and midwives, ignore it altogether. They think a glass or two of wine during pregnancy is fine. I was one of them. I was aware of the surgeon general's warnings, the social pressure not to drink, and the research, and this was my logic: The baby is most susceptible to neural and other birth defects in the first trimester. The brain is particularly vulnerable in the early weeks, when its basic structure is being formed; after this point, it is relatively well protected until middle pregnancy, when there is a massive growth spurt.[6] So I gave up wine for the first three months. Or nearly—I know I had a glass here and there. As it happened, I had almost no desire for wine, which may suggest some innate bodily wisdom. After that, I felt the baby was well on its way, that I was well nourished in general, and that the odd glass of wine, taken with food to absorb it, wouldn't hurt.

Drinking in public with a large, round belly may well attract funny looks from your fellow Americans. Oddly enough, I met with little criticism. More often, and to my surprise, people cheered me on. One summer night, I was noticeably pregnant and teaching a class on organic and biodynamic foods with a French winemaker at Murray's Cheese. I joined in on the wines. After class, a grandmother, proudly Italian, whispered in my ear, "Good for you, having a glass of wine. We all did. I told my daughter she ought to, but she wouldn't hear of it." She was not the only one.

For many pregnant women, not drinking is not an issue. They wouldn't dream of picking up a drink, any more than they would get stoned or take up cigarettes. Abstaining altogether is a great decision. Nine dry months seemed like a long time to me. (When Rose and Jacob were four, I pretty much quit, mostly to improve my mood.)

If you drink, you might limit yourself to one or two glasses of beer or wine a week, which amounts to light drinking by any measure. If you do choose to drink, there is no need to don a wig and sunglasses.

## GREEN IN THE GILLS

In April, I flew to Burlington, Vermont, to see my friend from Oberlin College, Caroline. She and her husband, Mike, had a toddler, Parker, and a new baby, Eliza Jane. I was about fourteen weeks pregnant, and looking for a glimpse of family life in all its joy and mess, plus some sisterly advice about mothering—not that I have been very good about taking advice, sisterly or otherwise. We went for a walk along the shore of Lake Champlain and looked across the water to the Adirondacks. It was brisk and I was cheerful. Suddenly I felt a little funny. I got down on all fours, put my cheek near the moist spring earth, and felt a little better. Then I threw up behind a tree.

Caroline shot me a sympathetic, knowing look. I almost thought I saw her suppress a little smile—not unkind exactly, just . . . remembering. But I didn't think being pregnant had anything to do with being sick. I figured I was the only one who'd eaten an egg for breakfast. *The eggs must be off*, I thought. By lunchtime I was myself again.

In torrid July, when I was five or six months pregnant, I was in Philadelphia on a book tour. I'd been up late with my hosts at the White Dog Cafe, a pioneering local food joint, and had to meet an early train, so I didn't have breakfast—just my vitamins. I put my bag in a taxi, but before climbing in, I turned and ran for the lobby restrooms, where I lost my fish oil. Yuck. Still, I didn't think being pregnant had anything to do with being sick. *I had a big dinner*, I thought. *I'm exhausted. It's hot.*

A few weeks later in Seattle, I jogged over to Pike Place Market to buy breakfast. Back in my hotel, I was chatting over Washington cherries with my friend Laura Cooper when I started to feel odd. No more cherries. Soon after, I was gustily eating superb Vietnamese food at a tiny spot called the Green Leaf with my friend Judy Amster, who is an exemplary guide to Seattle eating. After scoffing dessert, I got on a ferry and bobbed across Puget Sound to Bainbridge Island to another book event, feeling great.

Later it dawned on me that I was like many other pregnant women (imagine that) and that throwing up was baby-related. I thought I'd escaped the weird, unexplained nausea that plagues so many women, and furthermore, I smugly assumed it was because I was so healthy. Wrong on both counts.

All over the world, most women—60 to 75 percent—experience some nausea and vomiting in pregnancy, or NVP, as it's now called. Women in traditional and industrial cultures, North and South, East and West, complain of it. In the deserts of Botswana, !Kung women suffer, as do Japanese, Arab, European, and South African women. NVP is remarkably consistent, or, put another way, free of the patterns that make medical sleuthing rewarding. In traditional societies, there is no relationship between NVP and farming practices, work habits, social structure, community size, or settlement patterns. Black and white South Africans have similar rates of NVP. In short, NVP appears to be indifferent to region, lifestyle, race, and class.[7]

In other ways, NVP isn't consistent at all. Despite the term "morning sickness," it strikes day and night. It mars first pregnancies but not second ones, and vice versa. Nausea bothers women who eat junk food and women who don't. As I discovered with Julian, it may last well into the second trimester. With Rose and Jacob, I was nauseated and throwing up for thirty-eight weeks.

Symptoms of NVP include fatigue, nausea, queasiness, vomiting daily or several times daily, gag reflexes, dry heaves, powerful aversions, powerful cravings, the desire to eat something only to be disgusted by it, food indecision, overwhelming reactions to smells, a bad or metallic taste in the mouth, heartburn, and overactive salivary glands, also known as drooling.

The diagnosis hasn't changed. In the second century A.D., the Greek gynecologist, obstetrician, and pediatrician Soranus of Ephesus, author of *On Midwifery and the Diseases of Women*, which set medical opinion on children's and women's health for fifteen hundred years, listed these symptoms of pregnancy: "a stomach which is upset, indeed full of fluid; nausea and want of appetite, sometimes for all, sometimes for certain foods . . . appetite for things not customary like earth, charcoal, tendrils of the vine, unripe and acid fruit; excessive saliva, malaise, [belching] . . ."

Medical treatment for NVP hasn't changed, either. Soranus recommended fasting, eating small amounts of easily digested food, porridge, soft-boiled eggs, weak wine, massage, and the punching bag. And that's about all we have to say to pregnant women today: Whatever makes you comfortable is the right thing to do. Our understanding of NVP is poor. It's probably hormonal. One or more of the thirty or so pregnancy hormones may cause NVP. Which one, no one knows. HCG—the hormone detected by the pregnancy test—is one suspect. So are progesterone, estrogen, thyroxine, and growth factors called activin and inhibin.

But these are merely proximate causes. What is the ultimate purpose, if any, of the nearly universal condition once called morning sickness? MacArthur fellow Margie Profet proposed that NVP protects the fetus from food-borne toxins, in particular those that can cause birth defects during organogenesis, which occurs in the first twelve weeks. That might explain why many pregnant women find strong and bitter flavors in food such as cabbage, mustard, pepper, and coffee repugnant. The toxins in these plants are meant to keep insects at bay. In large doses they can poison humans.

The good news is that most symptoms in most women recede after about three months. Perhaps more important, symptoms of NVP are very common in healthy pregnancies. "It is almost unheard of for a fetus to suffer adverse effects from morning sickness, *regardless* of the degree," says the obstetrician Lynn Friedman in the foreword to *The Morning Sickness Companion* by Elizabeth Kaledin. Women with severe NVP have fewer miscarriages, stillbirths, premature babies, and babies with heart defects.

There is one slim hint that nutrition can help. Adequate vitamin $B_6$ may prevent and treat NVP. Foods rich in vitamin $B_6$

include tuna, beef, chicken, liver, avocados, bananas, and whole grains. Whether it's just as good to take additional $B_6$ once you have NVP as to be well stocked beforehand, I don't know. If you don't get enough $B_6$ from food, try Brewer's yeast. If you can't even manage that, consider a pill. One $B_6$ supplement for women feeling queasy comes in a lozenge, which might make it more palatable. It contains twenty-five milligrams of $B_6$, a whopping 1250 percent of the RDA.

Ginger, a traditional folk remedy for upset stomach and nausea, can also help. Ginger has long been used to treat seasick sailors and patients postsurgery. *Obstetrics and Gynecology* reported that 250 milligrams of powdered ginger reduced the severity of NVP symptoms in 90 percent of the women who took it.[8] (Nearly 30 percent felt better on the placebo—not bad.)

As for what foods to eat when you're nauseated, just do what works. Eat what feels good and eat when you need to. Miriam Erick, a dietician who cares for women hospitalized for the only kind of NVP to worry about—hyperemesis gravidarum, or severe, prolonged vomiting—has found no consistent evidence for food cravings or aversions. Some women crave meat, while others can't bear it, and likewise for most food.[9]

You have just one goal: to eat the best foods you can. Try not to fall back on "white foods." If bland carbohydrate is all you can manage, make it a banana, a dried apricot, or an oatcake with a dab of raw honey. At least they contain potassium, iron, B vitamins, and fiber. In many ways, the body of a well-nourished woman is no match for the needs of the fetus. Even if you eat very little, the baby will ransack your body for the nutrients required. The baby may borrow from your stores, but you can always replenish them when your appetite returns. If you're not pregnant yet, now is a great time to build up reserves by eating well. And if you're already pregnant and feeling queasy, take heart. It will probably be over soon.

## RED MEAT IS IRONCLAD

Mothers and babies simply must have iron and have it right from the start. Low maternal iron levels and anemia are linked to poor placental growth, low birth weight, and premature birth. The all-important role of iron can be summed up in one stark fact: Deficiency compromises fetal growth.[10] This metal carries oxygen from the lungs to every cell in the body. Its other big role is to make blood. Blood volume increases by 50 percent during pregnancy. Blood feeds the placenta and uterine lining. Without large numbers of oxygen-rich red blood cells, your baby won't grow.

Vital as iron is, I don't agree with the common advice on iron and pregnancy. The Centers for Disease Control recommends every pregnant woman take thirty grams of iron daily, and if anemia is suspected, twice that. But when I was pregnant, I didn't take iron pills. Why not? They may not work, for one thing. We know that iron-poor conditions stunt fetal growth, but it's not clear that supplements increase birth weight.[11]

Now ponder a more fundamental objection. What if anemia—as defined—is not even a problem? The CDC considers a pregnant woman anemic when hemoglobin—the pigment in red blood cells—is below 11 ml/dg, and typically, doctors will prescribe iron supplements. But skeptics ask whether prescribing iron helps mothers and babies. One study found "lack of evidence that screening for anemia improves clinical maternal, fetal, or neonatal outcome."[12]

How can we explain these vexing findings? It could be quite simple. The diagnosis is wrong. The average healthy pregnant woman may have lower hemoglobin, but she is not anemic. Hemoglobin concentration as low as 9.0 ml/dg in pregnancy is normal, not pathological. It's a side effect of greater blood volume, which is not only normal but essential for a healthy pregnancy. According to the obstetrician Michel Odent, the CDC standards "confuse a transitory physiological response (blood dilution) and a disease (anemia)."[13] The pediatrician Lendon Smith agrees: "The widely seen drop in iron blood levels in pregnant women signifies good expansion of blood volume, not anemia."[14]

Contrary to the assumptions behind the CDC guidelines, a study of 150,000 women found that *lower* hemoglobin levels are associated with *higher* birth weight. But when hemoglobin doesn't fall—a sign that blood volume has not risen—the risk of preeclampsia, preterm birth, and low birth weight rises.[15] Iron is important, but looking at iron alone is misguided. As we'll see shortly, when we discuss preeclampsia, the obstetrician Tom Brewer established that the best prevention for these conditions is not taking iron but eating more protein.

There are also doubts about supplemental iron itself. Supplements and fortified foods contain inorganic iron salts, which are poorly absorbed compared with the iron in food. Inorganic iron also interferes with nutrients vital for fetal growth, including zinc. Without zinc, protein synthesis falters. Zinc deficiency can cause preeclampsia, low birth weight, miscarriage, and birth defects. Low zinc levels in the placenta are linked to low birth weight and small head size in babies.

A common side effect of supplemental iron is constipation. The reasons iron disturbs digestion are curious. Sharon Moalem, author of *Survival of the Sickest: The Surprising Connections Between Disease and Longevity*, is an expert on iron metabolism, and he explained it to me in memorable terms. Certain pathogens thrive on iron. When you take extra iron, these iron-loving bacteria multiply and prosper. Your intestines look like an algae-choked pond, says Moalem. "Nothing can pass through." Dr. Natasha Campbell-McBride, an expert on gut flora, agrees that supplements don't work. "Iron makes these bacteria grow stronger and does not remedy anemia," she writes.[16]

Some experts think that pregnant women in particular should not take iron. When you get a virus, the body withholds iron to prevent invading bacteria from enjoying an iron feast.[17]

Put another way, temporary anemia is the body's deliberate response to infection. You may recall that during pregnancy, immunity is slightly depressed. A natural decline in iron concentration helps protect pregnant women from infection. That's why pediatrician Lendon Smith calls lower iron levels "innately prophylactic." He concludes that "routine iron supplements in pregnancy are unnecessary and unwise except in genuine iron-deficiency anemia."

That condition turns out to be rare, especially in well-off countries. True iron-deficiency anemia is more common in places where the diet is chronically inadequate. Most Americans probably get enough iron in absolute terms. A more common cause of anemia is poor absorption of iron. Diets high in grain contribute to anemia because grain is iron-poor and phytic acid in grain blocks iron. Inadequate protein, copper, folate, and vitamins $B_6$ and C depress iron absorption. Vitamin $B_{12}$ deficiency causes a particular condition called pernicious anemia. It's more common in pregnancy because the placenta is actively draining $B_{12}$ for the baby.

Adelle Davis tells us that "even severe" anemia can be treated with food. The iron in meat, called "heme," is better absorbed than nonheme iron from plants.[18] A little heme iron even makes the iron in plants more available. Adding just fifty grams of pork to an iron-poor meal raises nonheme iron absorption significantly.[19]

For a straight hit of iron, eating red meat or liver is a sure bet. Clams, chicken liver, duck, and oysters are excellent sources. Fish, poultry, leaves, dried apricots, and unsulphured or blackstrap molasses are decent sources. Grains and dairy foods are not. It's also wise to eat iron-friendly foods, including fresh produce for folate and vitamin C, bananas for $B_6$, and any meat, milk, or eggs for $B_{12}$.

If you take a supplement, consider Brewer's yeast or Floradix, a liquid with organic iron in an absorbable form (ferrous gluconate) instead of inorganic iron.[20] Another option is taking ground liver capsules. If you're not anemic, don't take iron. The body does not excrete iron easily, and too much can be toxic.

When you think of iron, think of red. The iron oxide in earth yields a range of pigments, from scarlet to brick, ruby to rust. Iron is what makes blood and muscle red. Traditional lore in China, Italy, and elsewhere says what modern nutrition tells us: that eating red foods is good for the blood. It comes as no surprise that the red foods recommended—beef, lamb, pork, liver—are rich in protein, B vitamins, and zinc, not to mention the metal itself. Iron metabolism may be complex, but remembering what to eat need not be. Red meat is ironclad.

## MOTHER AND BABY IN THE SECOND TRIMESTER

For many women, the second trimester comes as a relief and a pleasure. Around the fourth month, you may feel quite different. If you were dead on your feet, you may have a bounce in your step. Nausea might be fading. Perhaps you're even starting to show.

When I was pregnant, every couple of weeks or so, I added a note to the letter I was writing my Little Baby.

> Until you were about ten weeks old—the midwife calls that twelve weeks pregnant—I was very, very sleepy. You were growing so fast, all you wanted me to do was sleep. After twelve weeks, I wasn't sleepy anymore. And I had a little bump, like an orange, in my belly. That was the first time I could feel or see you.

The excitement of the bump! The baby isn't microscopic anymore. If you weren't hungry before, the baby may be calling for more. You may want to eat more or need to snack. Not long after, I wrote:

> I'm fifteen weeks pregnant. You are like a grapefruit in my belly: round, smooth, taut like a drum. You seem a bit

hungrier now. When I finish my lunch of beef or fish or chicken and salad and nuts and cheese or yogurt and fruit or chocolate, you seem to say, "How about a piece of bread?"

Only a week later, at four months, I couldn't lie on my stomach on a hard surface because the grapefruit was in the way. I was very pleased. Finally, I had to wear my jeans low, and I felt like eating for two—the perks of pregnancy!

In the second trimester, you're building the baby's muscle and bone. Now is the time to eat plenty of protein and calcium. They are the bricks and mortar of babies. By the end of the sixth month, the baby's bony skeleton is fully formed from the calcium you provide. Everything else—the placenta, the baby's skin, muscle, and fingernails—is made of protein. There are only two ways the baby can get the necessary protein and calcium: from your own muscle and bone, or from your dinner.

Naturally you'll carry on taking cod liver oil and any other prenatal supplements you've chosen. At meals, you have two new assignments. First, eat some whole protein at every opportunity. The baby uses it daily, and your body cannot store it. Second, eat some calcium-rich foods every day. Don't neglect fats, and saturated fats in particular, to absorb the calcium. Whole milk, sour cream, cheddar cheese, and not-too-sweet ice cream are good choices. If you don't care for dairy, try chicken soup.

Weight gain should be slow and steady and stay that way, right to the end. A gain of twenty-five to thirty-five pounds over thirty-eight to forty-two weeks is right for most women. (Women having twins will gain more, and should.) There is wide variability in total weight gain among healthy mother-baby pairs. Some well-fed women gain more than thirty-five pounds, while other women gain less than twenty-five eating well. Both over- and undereating are undesirable. Women who gain too much weight don't help their babies and have trouble losing it later. But if you don't eat some extra calories, you will burn protein and fat for energy, effectively putting the baby on a low-protein and low-fat diet. Reducing the calories you need by one third means that half the protein you eat is burned for energy.[21] That protein never reaches the baby.

Where does the extra weight go? The placenta, a bigger uterus, amniotic fluid, extra blood, and bigger breasts add about fifteen pounds. The baby weighs six to eight pounds. The rest will be in the extra padding on your hips, thighs, and bottom, if not everywhere. In some circles, skinny mothers with tidy watermelon bumps are in fashion, but don't be swayed. The baby needs you to carry a little extra weight all over. You'll use it up later, when you're nursing.

Try to focus on eating well, not on your weight. If you must choose a target weight, make it a range, not one number, and don't weigh yourself frequently. When you shop, find clothes that fit you right now, not next week. I wore lots of cheap, pretty sundresses, but I did buy one pair of maternity jeans, the kind you can adjust. They were outlandishly expensive and worth every penny. They looked as good at twenty weeks as they did at forty.

Now that the baby is bigger and hungrier, you may have to pay a little more attention to keep blood sugar steady. To understand why stable blood sugar is important, imagine you're not pregnant. In the course of a day, blood glucose rises and falls. In healthy people, that's fine. You can get by without eating every fifteen minutes because the body has ways of keeping things level. If you run low on blood sugar, you can burn glycogen—stored glucose. If you go too long without eating, you burn fat and lose weight.

The unborn baby does not have these options. He cannot regulate his own blood sugar by calling on glycogen. He cannot raid the fridge or buy a banana. He relies instead on a continuous flow of glucose from your blood to the placenta. To guard against those moments when your last meal was too long ago, or you've suddenly used up all your fuel sprinting for the bus, the baby keeps your blood sugar slightly elevated *all the time*. In this manner he is continuously well fed.

Mildly elevated blood sugar in pregnancy, in other words, is normal. But many women don't know that. At prenatal visits, blood sugar is routinely screened. The idea is to detect diabetes, which can be risky for mother and baby. Excessive blood sugar produces an oversized yet malnourished baby. Such babies are said to be "sugar soaked" and have a higher risk of obesity and diabetes. In the prenatal screen, you drink a sugary solution, and your doctor or nurse watches the spike on blood sugar. Many perfectly healthy women fail this test. If blood sugar rises too much, you're diagnosed with "gestational diabetes."

"This diagnosis is useless," says Dr. Michel Odent, "because it merely leads to simple recommendations that should be given to all pregnant women," such as: don't eat sugar, choose whole grains, and get some exercise. A large study found that routine glucose screening resulted in 3 percent of the women being told they had gestational diabetes. The diagnosis did not change birth outcomes.[22]

Your goal is simple. Keep blood sugar steady by eating complex carbohydrates, not white flour and sugar. Because they don't cause blood sugar to spike, fat and protein make excellent snacks. If you eat some olive oil, cheese, or nuts with a piece of bread, the fat and protein will cushion the effects of carbohydrates on blood sugar. Many women find it helpful to eat small, frequent meals.

And now you can tell everyone why you're constantly reaching for a bag of nuts or piece of cheese. At last, everyone can see your bump. You have a certain status. Perfect strangers are ready to give up seats, carry bags, hold doors, and generally celebrate your state. I enjoyed the pointless predictions about the baby's sex from old ladies, cops, and construction workers speculating about the shape of my belly. "Carrying high—that's a boy!" It's all groundless folklore, but who cares? The number of people who simply said, "God bless you" as I walked by was astonishing. The world loves a pregnant woman.

## PRENATAL SCARE

On a bright warm Saturday in May, I went to a "Love Your Park" cleanup and gardening session at Petrosino Square, a little park in Nolita, a corner of New York that isn't quite Little Italy and isn't quite Chinatown, to talk to local residents about a food market I was going to open there. I was sixteen weeks pregnant and feeling wonderful. The druggy exhaustion was only a memory.

After the pansies were planted, I did my spiel on the market, passed out some flyers, and chatted up the locals. I was pleased to see mothers and babies, because they're good customers for local food. I sat in the sun next to another pregnant woman, and we talked, as pregnant women do, about due dates and prenatal visits.

Her experience and mine were quite different. I went to a midwife; she saw an obstetrician. That put me in a minority, at least in this country. In many industrialized countries, midwives attend about 70 percent of births, in homes, birth centers, and hospitals.[23] In the United States in 2013, midwives attended about 320,093 births (about 12 percent of vaginal births and 8 percent of all births), a figure that has been climbing steadily since 2004. I was also hoping to have the baby at home—"all being well," as I often added, not wishing to tempt fate. Here that's very rare. In 2012, just over 1 percent of American babies were born at home, compared with 20 percent of Dutch babies.

Women were sometimes uneasy when I mentioned home birth. "Not for me. I'd be too scared." That is a good reason not to do it. Mother and baby will probably have the best experience where the mother feels most secure. I wasn't intending to be fearless or foolish. I simply thought I'd be more comfortable at home—and equally safe. No doubt that's partly because I was born at home myself. It's also because I've read up on the statistics on home birth. The countries with the lowest infant mortality, such as Iceland, Finland, Norway, The Netherlands, and Japan, are those where midwifery is a routine part of obstetric care and home birth is not unusual.

On we went, gingerly addressing each pregnancy topic. My park-bench friend was getting ultrasounds at each doctor's visit; I hadn't and didn't plan to. She was getting amniocentesis, but I wasn't. I don't remember exactly what I said. "Yeah, I didn't really want to do amnio, either," she said. "But I had to, because I'm thirty-five. You know, Down syndrome."

I didn't say anything. I was thirty-five, too, and I was aware of the gradually rising risks of birth defects with AMA—the abbreviation for "advanced maternal age" they wrote on our charts. But I didn't consider my age alone sufficient grounds for getting a needle through my belly and uterus. I had no desire to question her choices, but once I found that our sensibility was poles apart, I didn't much want to explain mine, either. Many pregnant women feel the same. For fear of appearing critical and being judged, we keep mum.

This stalemate is lamentable. Decisions on prenatal testing and how you want to give birth are personal and delicate, but how much better if we could talk about them openly! If you're considering genetic screening, do read about the advantages and

## INFANT DEATHS

| | PER 1,000 LIVE BIRTHS, 2003[24] |
|---|---|
| United States (midwife-attended) | 2.1 |
| Singapore | 2.28 |
| Sweden | 2.77 |
| Netherlands | 5.11 |
| United Kingdom | 5.22 |
| United States (all births) | 6.3 |

disadvantages and talk to mothers who've been there. In *Gentle Birth, Gentle Mothering*, Dr. Sarah Buckley presents the pitfalls. In *Having Faith*, on the other hand, Sandra Steingraber gives a thoughtful account of her reasons for getting amniocentesis.

As for the birth itself, there are more choices than ever and many good ones. But one thing is sure. The march of technology into the birthing room has been steady. In a famous 1920 article and speech to his fellow obstetricians, Joseph DeLee declared (preposterously) that "labor is a pathological process," and recommended the routine use of episiotomy, forceps, and sedation by means of morphine, chloroform, ether, and scopolamine, an amnesiac drug. Drugs such as chloroform had been used in childbirth since the 1840s, but DeLee's comments gave a strong push to the medical and surgical revolution in birth. Thankfully, sedation and amnesia are part of the past, but ultrasound, amniocentesis, induction with synthetic hormones, epidurals, and episiotomy are routinely used in healthy women.

Cesarean rates in this country—about 30 percent of births each year from 2009 to 2014—are too high. According to the 2015 statement on cesarean sections from the World Health Organization, such a high rate of surgeries has no benefit. "At population level, caesarean section rates higher than ten percent are not associated with reductions in maternal and newborn mortality rates." Most experts agree that many, or at least some, of these cesareans are not medically necessary. Whether medically justified or not, cesareans also tend to beget more cesareans. According to the Listening to Mothers Survey, many women who would like a vaginal birth after a cesarean (VBAC) are unable to find a doctor willing to attend. That's unfortunate, because babies born via surgery are at higher risk of allergies, asthma, ADHD, autism, celiac disease, obesity, and Type 2 diabetes.

For me the choice was easy. I was hoping for a traditional birth. My midwife, Linda Perry, had, in her words, "caught" more than four hundred babies at home. She was a mother of six who would treat my pregnancy as a normal event in my life, not a medical one. I was prepared to embrace the mystery of carrying a baby, including its sex and DNA. Linda could use her hands to guess its size and position.

Another benefit of seeing a midwife was the gentle tone of the typical prenatal visit. Too often, these appointments revolve around the things that might go wrong. For some women, of course, things do go wrong. But for most healthy women, all is well. Unlike Dr. DeLee, Linda assumed that the peculiar things happening to me were normal, not pathological. You don't have a disease. You have a baby.

Dr. Odent is a surgeon and midwife who knows both sides of birth, the surgical and the traditional. Since the 1950s, he has performed many cesareans and attended many home births. In *The Cesarean*, Odent discusses the "prenatal scare."

> The modern pregnant woman cannot be blissfully happy. All of them have at least one reason to be worried: "Your blood pressure is too high or too low," "Your weight is increasing too quickly or too slowly," "You are anemic," "You might hemorrhage because your platelet count is low," "You have gestational diabetes," "Your baby is too small or too big," "There is too much liquid around the baby," "There is a lack of liquid," "The placenta is low," "You are 18 and teenage pregnancy is associated with specific risks," "You are 39 and older-age pregnancy is associated with specific risks," "Your baby has not yet turned head-first," "The baby's back is on the right side, which makes the birth difficult," "According to the blood sample you are at risk of having a Down's syndrome baby," "You did not take folic acid at the right time and we must consider the risk of spina bifida," "You are not immunized against rubella," "You are rH negative," "If you have not given birth on Wednesday, we must consider an induction," etc.

Ideally, prenatal visits are boring. Apart from the stethoscope and scale, no machines need be involved. It's quite normal for nothing at all to happen. The main activity is talking, and the most important question, *How are you feeling?*

The doctors don't mean to frighten us, of course. Each of the conditions Odent mentions can indeed affect the health of mother and baby. It's just that in most healthy women, they don't. A worried doctor makes for a worried woman. Perhaps the reverse is true, too. The woman worries her doctor. Goodness knows, pregnant women in the United States are worried. In *Deliver This! Make the Childbirth Choice That's Right for You . . . No Matter What Everyone Else Thinks*, Marisa Cohen writes:

> Most of us spend our entire pregnancies in constant fear that something will go wrong . . . I dutifully read *What To Expect When You're Expecting*, which in its overarching, informative style, talked about every possible thing that could go terribly wrong . . . In my sixth and seventh month, I would check BabyCenter.com every week or so to see what the odds were of my baby surviving if she were born that day . . . I considered myself one of the more *relaxed* pregnant women I knew.

Anxiety is the enemy of an easy pregnancy, a smooth birth, and poised motherhood. In other cultures, being relaxed is understood as the proper state for a mother-to-be. In ancient China, women practiced Tai-kyo, meaning "embryonic education" or "womb learning." The essence of Tai-kyo, which has also been practiced in Japan for four centuries, is that a happy and healthy woman has a healthy baby.[25] In the United States, Tai-kyo is invoked to encourage women to play Mozart against their bellies to ensure that Junior is a genius. Fathers are to speak regularly into the bump. I don't wish to be unkind, but this interpretation of Tai-kyo seems distorted. By all means, laugh, sing, and play piano when you're pregnant, and yes—talk to your unborn baby. We did. (Who wouldn't?) But don't be systematic.

Worry is more than a waste of time, a nuisance, psychological clutter. Anxiety increases the production of stress hormones, such as cortisol, which inhibits protein synthesis and antibody production.[26] Fear also raises the level of adrenaline, which suppresses oxytocin, the hormone of contractions and mother love. Lack of oxytocin makes for a longer, more difficult labor. It makes breast-feeding trickier and delays bonding with your baby.

When you find yourself pregnant, think carefully about who will look after you and the baby. Your doctor or midwife should make you feel calm and secure. Later, when you go into labor, have only those people who make you relaxed nearby. Nervous types, control freaks, and scaredy-cats don't get an invitation. They have too much adrenaline, and it's contagious. Your goal is simple: Keep *your* adrenaline down, which allows your body to produce the hormones you need, when you need them.

## AN OUNCE OF PREVENTION

I was paying for photos at the drugstore when the cover story on a weekly glossy caught my eye. A Hollywood actress, pregnant with twins, was said to be suffering from swelling, high blood pressure, and fainting. Everyone was worried, and medics were standing by. Later, doctors diagnosed preeclampsia and put her in the hospital on bed rest until the babies were deemed big enough to be delivered by cesarean. Preeclampsia is characterized by sudden and severe swelling, hypertension, and protein in the urine. It typically occurs late in pregnancy, and it's dangerous for mother and baby.

Now, I had no idea if these reports were true, and if they were, why she wasn't well, but I found myself wondering if the mother-to-be had been eating real food and enough of it. She's known for being skinny and for working hard. If a pregnant friend of mine told me she had these symptoms, I'd want to know about her diet. Protein is powerful in pregnancy, more powerful than you might think. According to the groundbreaking, but sadly underappreciated, research of the obstetrician Tom Brewer—work he did back in the 1970s—preeclampsia is caused by protein deficiency.

To understand why, first consider a healthy pregnancy. A little swelling is normal. Estrogen causes you to retain fluid in the tissues; as we've mentioned, blood volume increases significantly to feed the placenta. This extra blood has a noticeable side effect: slightly elevated blood pressure. That's normal, too. "An isolated increased blood pressure is usually a good sign of placental activity," writes Michel Odent in *The Farmer and the Obstetrician*. "The placenta—as the advocate of the baby—manipulates maternal physiology via the release of hormones and asks the mother to provide more blood." Mild hypertension in pregnancy is associated with good outcomes for mother and baby.

Sometimes swelling is unpleasant. Bulging hands and feet are unsightly and painful—a nuisance at best. At worst, it's the first symptom of preeclampsia. If you don't eat enough protein, the liver cannot manufacture sufficient protein to circulate in your blood. One of the most common proteins in blood is albumin. Its job is to hold water and salt inside your blood vessels—where they belong—so that fluid doesn't leak into your tissues. When albumin gets too low, you puff up. The same thing happens in extreme malnutrition. The distended bellies of starving children are caused by severe protein deficiency, a condition called kwashiorkor.

Brewer found that protein deficiency caused poor placental growth, swelling, preeclampsia, and premature birth, and then he set about preventing it. The Brewer diet calls for one hundred grams of high-quality protein from meat, poultry, fish, eggs, and milk daily. (Twins need another thirty grams.) Adelle Davis, another fan of protein in pregnancy, calls for seventy-five to one hundred grams.

Perhaps you're surprised at these high numbers—I was. But it's not too difficult to follow this advice. Three or four ounces of beef, pork, poultry, or fish—a modest serving—contains twenty to twenty-five grams of protein. To satisfy Davis, you need to eat four or five small servings of meat or fish. That's manageable, and you may be relieved to find out that most portions contain more than three ounces. When I was pregnant, my lunch was often a whole can of wild salmon, which provides forty-five grams of protein. With a meal like that, you're halfway there.

Brewer did much of his work in health clinics in the American South, treating women eating protein-poor diets made up of grits, black-eyed peas, okra, biscuits, and fatback. He had to recommend affordable, quality protein, so a quart of milk and two eggs daily made up the foundation of his diet. A cup of milk or yogurt has eight or nine grams of protein, an egg six or seven. To get a hundred grams of protein from milk, you'd have to drink more than ten glasses, which is probably more than most women would enjoy. Still, the doctor's confidence in milk and eggs is good news if you're a vegetarian or on a tight budget.

If you're an omnivore, eat the whole chicken, with skin and bones, not merely the meat. This ensures you'll get enough of two important amino acids, glycine and methionine. Glycine is vital for protein synthesis. Usually, you make enough to meet daily needs, but in pregnancy you need more. Glycine, which is found in skin and bones, is the "limiting factor" for protein synthesis in the baby.[27] That means there is no good substitute if you run out. Methionine, meanwhile, is found in muscle. It's also important, but methionine depletes glycine, so if you eat only muscle and leave the skin, the baby will be short of glycine. If you don't care for the skin on a roast chicken, proper beef or chicken stock provides glycine.

Don't rely on soy for protein. Vegetarian mothers are five times more likely to give birth to a boy with hypospadias—a common birth defect—than omnivores. "Soy is the likeliest culprit as no other commonly eaten food is high in phytoestrogens," writes Kaayla T. Daniel in *The Whole Soy Story*.[28]

If you struggle to eat enough meat, fish, and eggs, I can suggest a traditional supplement. Whey has the highest "biological value" of any known protein, which simply means your body uses it well. Whey is so nutritious, people raise pigs on it. Human nutritional needs are very similar to a pig's. Whey is handy because it's liquid and digestible. When the baby starts to squash your stomach against your rib cage, it's nice to know there's a light and drinkable protein made of real food.

When I first read about protein and preeclampsia, I did feel a little fretful. I wasn't sure I could eat a hundred grams of protein every day, and the consequences of eating too little were a bit harrowing. I soon got over it. After working out a few numbers (such as the protein in a can of fish) to get the general idea, I never counted protein again. I'm sure I often ate less than one hundred grams of protein in one day—probably much less. Yet I never had any swelling, the first sign of missing protein.

This is what I gathered from the research in Brewer's riveting book, *What Every Pregnant Woman Should Know*, and what I hope you'll remember: Eating ample protein is important, and it's safe to eat as much as you want. In *The Fertility Diet*, Jorge Chavarro, Walter C. Willett, and Patrick J. Skerrett say that eating up to 125 grams of protein daily is "perfectly reasonable" for healthy people. You won't overdose. Remember that protein is not stored. When you eat more protein than you need, you just pee it out.

One more thing: It's fine to salt your food freely. Obstetricians used to tell women who complained of swelling to sharply restrict salt. Unfortunately, this bad advice won't go away. I heard it from a yoga instructor. Half the class had swollen ankles, and she told us to cut out salt and drink more water. Yet salty foods are permitted on traditional prenatal diets (in Vietnam, for example) because pregnant women have special needs for salt. Blood and amniotic fluid are briny. If you restrict salt, blood volume is too low. The placenta may fail to grow, parts of it can die, and it may separate from the uterus. All these things threaten fetal growth.

Use as much unrefined sea salt as you want, in the kitchen and on the table, but avoid canned foods made with pure sodium chloride. Buy unsalted canned tomatoes and rinse canned chickpeas. Eat plenty of fresh produce for potassium, which should be in balance with sodium. Don't think about how much salt you're eating. Just drink to thirst and salt to taste. If you start to swell up, eat more steak and eggs. It sounds funny, I know, but it's true. With Rose and Jacob, I got preeclampsia, so I know all about it.

## THE DAY I FORGOT I WAS PREGNANT

Folk wisdom says that you lose one tooth with each pregnancy. There's probably some truth in it; a woman with weak bones gets pregnant, and the baby robs her body of the minerals it can. She nurses, gets pregnant again, and more minerals literally dissolve, vanish. "During pregnancy and nursing, calcium is pulled from bone if not adequate in the diet. The fetus and the mammary gland will not be denied." So says my friend Joann Grohman, a dairy farmer and expert in cow and human nutrition.

In the second trimester, your job is to eat lots of calcium to build your baby's bones and teeth. That much we agree on. The interesting question is how to get the calcium you need. As with iron, I didn't take supplements when I was pregnant. The calcium in tablets is often poorly absorbed, which may be why supplemental calcium doesn't always improve outcomes for mother and baby.[29] We've mentioned that you need fat, especially saturated fat, to absorb calcium. Brewer agrees that without fat, "calcium will not be assimilated."

In the traditional American diet, you can't beat whole milk for calcium. It contains vitamins A and D and saturated fats, essential partners for calcium. Women who eat less dairy when pregnant have babies with more tooth decay.[30] I found this astonishing, until I learned that the baby's teeth begin to form in the fifth month of pregnancy.

Real milk is best, of course. According to the prenatal diet researcher Amanda Rose, there is more available calcium in fermented dairy foods than fresh.[31] In other words, cheese, yogurt, sour cream, and crème fraîche provide more calcium than a glass of milk. Raw milk offers more calcium than pasteurized because the enzyme phosphatase, which you need to absorb calcium, is rendered ineffective by the heat used in pasteurization.

When I was pregnant, raw milk was heaven-sent, especially in the first weeks. When I wasn't hungry for any food at all, raw milk was hydrating, nutritious, and good for my digestion. The benefits of raw milk are well understood, but is it safe? I have read pages and pages on this topic and discussed it with many experts, from dairy farmers to raw-food advocates to food safety regulators. Long before I got pregnant, this is what I wrote in *Real Food*.

> Is raw milk safe? Like vegetables or meat, milk can be contaminated with pathogens, but raw milk is not inherently more susceptible than pasteurized milk or any other food. Clean raw milk from a healthy cow, carefully handled by a conscientious farmer, is safe. Safety starts in the dairy. Crowded, poorly fed, and weak herds are more susceptible to disease. The cow's ideal habitat is outdoors, her best diet grass. The careful farmer avoids contamination from pathogens by using clean buckets, strainers, and other equipment. Milk must be rapidly chilled after milking and kept cold. If you fancy raw milk, find a sparkling clean dairy—ideally one you can visit—with healthy, grass-fed cows and a farmer who drinks raw milk. The best choice is a certified dairy, where the cows are regularly tested for tuberculosis and brucellosis.

I didn't explain at length how many cases of pathogenic bacteria are found in pasteurized milk compared to certified raw milk—either total cases or cases per serving, although you can look this up if you are statistically inclined. I didn't dismantle the FDA's charges against raw milk or cite studies behind the rebuttals. I didn't trace the illnesses blamed on raw dairy to show how many more people get sick from pasteurized milk and cheese. I could have done all these things, but others have done it better.

Instead, I relied on an argument from common sense, and I'll do something like that here. Pathogens can and do enter the food supply at any point—before, during, or after pasteurization, packaging, cooking, and serving. Some, like *Listeria monocytogenes* and *E. coli*, can make you sick—usually temporarily, with a bout of what people delicately call intestinal distress. In rare cases, these pathogens cause fatal complications, usually in people with weakened immunity. Thus, my general rule: When you eat traditional foods, make sure you find a source you trust. For me that logic, and the data I've based it on, was good enough.

Then I got pregnant. Pregnancy is a different story. This is what you need to know. Listeriosis, the disease caused by *Listeria*, is relatively rare and usually not severe. Many cases are mild, but some are fatal. You are slightly more susceptible to *Listeria* when pregnant. Worse, listeriosis can cause miscarriage, prematurity, and infection or death in the newborn. Some prenatal cases are treated with antibiotics, but the main thing is to not eat *Listeria*. The American Pregnancy Association recommends avoiding deli meat that hasn't been properly reheated, pâté, smoked seafood, soft cheese, raw-milk cheese, and of course, raw milk itself. These foods can and do carry *Listeria*.

All this I knew, and I intended to avoid cheap deli meats and other industrial foods likely to be contaminated, as I generally do. I also intended to eat aged raw milk cheeses and soft cheeses, as many pregnant Europeans do. What I wasn't sure about was drinking raw milk, however much I trusted the dairy farmer and the creamery.

On Saturday, February 18, I was in London visiting my farmers' markets. It was cold and rainy. I had known I was pregnant for only four days, and already I was preternaturally sleepy, physically exhausted, constipated, and not at all hungry. But I also needed to eat *something*. At the market in Twickenham, I came upon the dairy stall selling green-top milk, the name for untreated milk in England. The perfect, digestible snack. I bought a pint, drank it down, and felt altogether better as I bid farewell to the market manager and boarded a train heading back to central London to catch the play *A Man for All Seasons*.

Then I remembered that I was pregnant, that I wasn't sure about raw milk, that I meant to do some more homework about the odds of getting listeriosis and the odds of a very unhappy outcome for the baby and me.

Yup. That's how it happened. *I forgot I was pregnant.* Which is a great joke on me, because my diary on February 15—one day after I peed on the stick—says, "almost already used to the idea of being pregnant." That evening at the opera, head full of baby thoughts, I found it difficult to concentrate on *Rigoletto*. At the intermission, I scribbled names on the program. Only three days later, I'd forgotten I was going to have a baby.

Eventually, of course, I did my homework, and as you know, I decided to drink raw milk right through my forty weeks. It was right for me, but you will have to make up your own mind. If you examine the arguments for raw milk closely, you'll probably feel pretty sure either way. Meanwhile, it goes without saying that large numbers of healthy babies are born to mothers who drink pasteurized milk. I drank plenty myself and still do. Just buy the best milk you can.

If you don't care for dairy foods, or find it hard to eat large amounts for any reason, broth is the best source of calcium. Vietnamese believe that a gelatinous broth made from tiger bones gives you strong bones. Stock contains minerals in a form the body can easily absorb, and not only calcium, but also magnesium, phosphorus, silicon, sulphur, and trace minerals. The minerals emerge when you boil bones for a long time with a little acid, such as wine or lemon juice. Another excellent source of calcium is canned salmon, if you eat the tiny bones. I often ate it when I was pregnant. It's convenient and affordable pantry food, and it packs calcium, protein, and omega-3 fats in one easy dose. I do not recommend imitation milk made from soybeans for calcium. Phytic acid in soy blocks calcium.

## MOTHER AND BABY IN THE THIRD TRIMESTER

By now you're used to being pregnant. You know that it's not a fixed condition. It's fluid, changeable. But one thing is going inexorably in one direction. Your belly gets bigger and bigger. As fit as you may be, everyone gets a little clunkier in the third trimester. Perhaps you're dragging a bit. When you're nine months pregnant, time may be dragging, too. By my definition, "nine months pregnant" is the period from thirty-six weeks until the Birth Day, which may span six weeks, if the baby is two weeks "late." Days can be long. Nights, too. The baby's head sits on your bladder, urging you constantly to pee. Sitting may be awkward, not to mention standing, sleeping, car trips, shopping, and any other position or activity you care to mention.

*Bon courage!* No one stays pregnant forever. You're near the end. And if this is your first baby, these are magical, never-to-be-repeated weeks. It's much easier to carry a seven or eight pounder in your belly than to look after one outside it. Right now, his breathing, eating, drinking, peeing, and pooping are taken care of automatically. He doesn't squirm out of your arms, and you can't drop him. He doesn't need clothes and can't get frostbite or sunburn. You have the use of two hands. You sleep at will, or close enough. You wash your hair often. You go to movies and eat at restaurants. Later, when you find yourself in an altogether different universe, New Motherland, you may remember all this. Perhaps you will marvel at the efficiency and tidiness of pregnancy.

At the end, my chief complaint had to do with my line of work and my stubborn nature. I knew too much, but I was fed up with eating properly. My stomach was squished against my ribs, which demanded smaller meals, but I hate "grazing" and nibbling. I was tired of rib eye and lamb. I wanted ice cream and wine. Sometimes I had both, the first at four P.M. and the other at seven. But I was too Goody Two-shoes to give in completely to junk food. On October 9, I wrote my friend Joann Grohman— mother of eight, grandmother of sixteen, great-grandmother of four—to complain.

> Thirty-eight weeks. Today I said the hell with protein and made brown rice, miso soup, and sliced pickled cucumbers. I suppose I am a little weary of eggs, meat, fish, and cheese at every meal, and miss my occasional girl's suppers of all salad. I did put two great big tablespoons of grass-fed butter on the rice. Give me points: My stomach is the size of Hunca Munca's and I feel I could eat from doll's dishes.

I had been reading a life of Beatrix Potter; hence the reference to her character Hunca Munca, the naughty mouse who moves into a dollhouse and wrecks the place. Joann, a nutrition maven, can be strict about these things. I smiled when I read her reply: "Eat whatever you want."

Of course there are reasons to eat well—bingeing on sugar won't help—but do give yourself a get-out-of-jail-free pass occasionally. You can certainly relax about nutrients for organ development. You've pretty much built your baby. There's no reason to start eating junk food willy-nilly, but it's more than merely tolerable if you don't get the perfect array of prenatal foods every day, or even over two or three days—it's inevitable.

If you're tempted to give in and eat garbage, there are good reasons not to. The baby's skeleton is fully formed by six months or so, but the bones themselves bulk up dramatically in the last three months, so keep eating calcium. Babies born six weeks premature have half the calcium in their bones of full-term babies.[32] Keep eating oysters and beef for zinc. You will transfer a massive dose of zinc to the baby in the last ten weeks, right up to the days before birth, which is why premature babies can be deficient in zinc. Keep eating meat, dairy, and eggs for protein and vitamin $B_{12}$. In the last two months you begin to transfer $B_{12}$ to your baby. Deficiency of $B_{12}$ causes prematurity. The protein will prevent swelling, which can get worse at the end. Finally, keep drinking water. The baby needs plenty of amniotic fluid. Dehydration is a common cause of premature labor.

Fat is the main thing in the third trimester. The baby is putting on subcutaneous fat, so she's not born too skinny. In newborns, fat has three purposes. It's an energy reserve, in case your milk takes a while to come in or production temporarily runs short of demand. Second, it insulates her body. Third, a special fat at the back of her neck, called brown fat, will actually burn "hot," warming her body itself.

Getting fat is easy. Your baby can put on body fat from any food you eat. Donuts made with white flour and trans fats will do it, and so will steak and baked potato. But there is only one place to get the fully formed EPA and DHA she needs to build her big, fat *Homo sapiens* brain, and that is fish. If you're not eating it, you're giving it away. Your personal omega-3 stores decrease steadily during pregnancy, as the baby siphons off the fat she needs. The transfer of DHA, in particular, increases sharply in the third trimester to feed the fetal brain.[33] You are also storing omega-3 fats to make milk. Babies born too early lack extra fat, so they're more dependent on your milk for omega-3 fats.

As you waddle through these final days, feeling like a hippopotamus one day and a seal the next, remember who you are. I mean deep down, back through the mists of evolutionary time. You are an aquatic ape. Now more than ever, it's time to act like the water-loving mammal you are. Go ahead—perform like a seal. Eat plenty of fish, so your baby can build her brain made of fat.

## BRAIN FOOD

Filipinos believe that fish head soup is brain food, and they are right. Brain cell membranes are made of fats called phospholipids, which account for one quarter of solid brain matter. The most abundant fats in brain cells by far are the very long-chain omega-3 fatty acid DHA and the very long-chain omega-6 fatty acid known as arachidonic acid (ARA). In the last trimester, your baby's brain grows by four- or fivefold.[34] Together, DHA and ARA fuel the growth spurt.

ARA is found in meat, eggs, and milk. There is every reason to eat pork chops and cheddar cheese in the last trimester, but chances are you will get enough ARA without trying. ARA is in many common foods, and you can also make some from another omega-6 oil, linoleic acid (LA), which is abundant in nuts and seeds. But do make an effort to get DHA, which you'll find in fish. There's a wee bit in grass-fed meat and pastured eggs, but seafood is simply the best way to get the DHA your baby needs.

By all means, eat fish throughout your pregnancy, but do pile it on at the end. Another benefit of eating seafood is iodine. Severe deficiency causes cretinism, a neurological disorder. That's not likely, but there is evidence that moderate deficiency causes milder mental problems.[35] You will also need fish to make milk rich in DHA and to prevent postnatal depression. If that weren't enough, the benefits of omega-3 fats extend beyond the brain. Eating plenty of fish now will help prevent premature labor and low birth weight.

As we've seen, seafood may contain methylmercury, which causes brain damage, learning difficulties, and poor motor skills in children. In 2004, the U.S. government advised women trying to conceive and pregnant women not to consume more than 340 grams of seafood per week, to avoid possible mental damage from methylmercury. That's twelve ounces, or about two six-ounce portions a week. Caution is sensible, but some experts think that we've been a little too successful at steering pregnant women away from fish.

Dr. Michel Odent, the prenatal nutrition expert, countered that the benefits of fish to mother and baby are "enormous."[36] In 2005, researchers at the Harvard School of Public Health announced that the mercury warnings could cause a pregnant woman to eat too little fish, not only for the baby's brain but also for her own health.[37]

The official advice probably did make women scared to eat fish. In 2007, Joseph Hibbeln, an expert on omega-3 fats at the National Institutes of Health, published a study of more than eleven thousand pregnant women near Bristol, England. The women consumed varying degrees of seafood each week: none at all, around the recommended limit of 340 grams, or more than 340 grams, which came to about three servings a week. Researchers later assessed the women's children, aged six months to eight years, for various measures of mental and social development. Even after accounting for about two dozen confounding factors, including social disadvantage, perinatal health, and other aspects of diet, the children of women eating less than two servings of fish per week had lower verbal, fine motor, and social skills than the children of the fish-eating mothers. For every outcome measured, the lower the seafood intake, the higher the chances of poor development in the kids. The researchers concluded:

> Maternal seafood consumption of less than 340 grams per week in pregnancy did not protect children from adverse outcomes; rather, we recorded beneficial effects on child development with maternal seafood intakes of more than 340 grams per week, suggesting that advice to limit seafood consumption could actually be detrimental. These results show that risks from the loss of nutrients were greater than the risks of harm from exposure to trace contaminants in 340 grams seafood eaten weekly.[38]

The team found "no evidence to lend support to the warnings of the U.S. advisory that pregnant women should limit their seafood consumption." The Bristol study didn't even ask whether the women were eating fish low or high in methylmercury. It found that eating more fish was better for babies, period. This and other data showing no harm from high prenatal fish consumption have led some researchers to ask whether fish could even *protect* against toxic methylmercury.[39] Furthermore, selenium binds with methylmercury. Most popular fresh and ocean fish (except swordfish) contain more selenium than methylmercury. That reduces the dose of the toxin.

In 2014, the FDA and EPA, citing evidence that fish is important for fetal development, early infancy in breastfed babies, and childhood, issued new draft advice to women who may become pregnant, pregnant and lactating women, and children: Eat eight to twelve ounces of a variety of fish that are relatively low in mercury.

Don't avoid fish, just methylmercury. Steer clear of bigger, older, and more carnivorous fish, including swordfish, shark, king mackerel, or tilefish. Don't eat sushi-grade tuna more than twice a week. The cautious pregnant woman might prefer to avoid tuna, a large carnivore, altogether. I ate lots of canned tuna myself. It's affordable and convenient, and I happen to love salade niçoise, a sterling prenatal dish. If you like canned tuna, look for brands selling line-caught albacore from clean Pacific waters, such as American Tuna or Vital Choice. These are younger and smaller than other tuna. The small, fatty fish, like anchovy, pilchard, herring, and common mackerel, are very safe. Mostly herbivorous fish such as catfish, carp, trout, and tilapia are also good choices.

I love all seafood, but my very favorite fish—and top baby food—is wild salmon. A 3.5-ounce (100-gram) portion of wild sockeye salmon contains more than 1,200 milligrams of omega-3 fats. Cold-water, oily fish (mackerel, herring, bluefish, salmon) have more omega-3 fats than the white, flaky fish. It's sensible to eat fatty fish two or three times a week. When you do cook fish, be generous with butter or cream. Saturated fats extend the supply of omega-3 fats; hence classics like Dover sole with butter sauce, lobster claws in butter, and creamy clam chowder.

You can also take a good fish oil supplement, such as Vital Choice or Nordic Naturals. Do not depend on cod liver oil for omega-3 fats. Cod liver oil contains large amounts of vitamins A and D, but only few omega-3 fats. Fish oil, by contrast, contains large amounts of omega-3 fats, but scant vitamins.

By urging you to eat plenty of fish in pregnancy, I don't mean to defend methylmercury. It's very dangerous to babies and children. Methylmercury poisoning causes problems with thinking, language, memory, motor skills, perception, and behavior. It's a poison best avoided. Just don't toss all fish overboard. Eat clean fish instead.

## NOT A TAX RETURN

My baby was due on October 24. I wrote "forty weeks" in my diary, but I tried not to focus on the date itself. When people asked when I was due, I said, "in late October." Doctors are obsessed with due dates. If your baby is "late," they threaten to induce labor. That makes women nervous. They take castor oil and get acupuncture, practice yoga and do water aerobics, in order to get the baby out before the doctor says he'll do it himself, something doctors often do. In the 1980s, induction with synthetic oxytocin, which is made from the pituitary glands of mammals, became the norm for any healthy woman pregnant past forty-two weeks.

Where did we get the idea that pregnancy lasts forty weeks? In the early 1800s, a German obstetrician, Franz Carl Naegele, declared human gestation to last ten lunar months. At twenty-eight days apiece, that came to 280 days, or forty weeks. But this is only an estimate, and probably a bit short. The average first pregnancy actually lasts forty-one weeks and three days, or 290 days.[40] Second babies tend to come a week sooner, after 283 days.[41] Of course these numbers cannot forecast your baby's Birth Day. It must be stressed that they are averages.

Even if 280 days were the average period babies spend in the womb, the numbers are skewed by about two weeks because, if you've paid close attention, doctors don't start counting from conception. They count from the first day of your last period, which is roughly two weeks *before* conception. They don't want to rely on when you think you conceived. Even if you think you know, sperm can survive for up to five days inside you before the mature egg arrives to be fertilized. Despite our attempts at precision, biology has soft edges.

Very few babies—about 5 percent—are born on the predicted due date. The vast majority—about 80 percent—are born between thirty-eight and forty-two weeks.[42] Your baby will almost certainly be one of them. Five to 10 percent of pregnancies go to forty-two weeks, the official marker of "postdate," and most of these babies turn out fine.[43]

Just as some babies sit up straight at four months and some at six, babies are born when they're ready. That's why inducing labor merely because forty-two weeks have passed is medically contentious. The *American Family Physician* calls it "controversial."[44] Unfortunately, it's also common. About 80 percent of women in American hospitals receive drugs to begin or to hasten labor.[45] But the American College of Obstetricians and Gynecologists opposes inducing labor in healthy women. ACOG policy says that inducing labor should be reserved for medical conditions such as preeclampsia.

We don't know exactly what triggers labor, but all evidence points to the baby, not the calendar. "The baby initiates labor by sending endocrine signals to the placenta," writes Sheila Kitzinger in *The Complete Book of Pregnancy and Childbirth*. These hormones prompt the baby's lungs to mature. "If labor is induced artificially, the timing may not be right either for the uterus to work most effectively or for the baby to be ready."[46] Curiously, these signals are stress hormones. Adrenaline and noradrenaline surge before labor. Writes Kitzinger:

> They protect the baby from a shortage of oxygen, shunt blood away from nonessential organs—the skin, for example—ensure a rich supply of blood to the heart, brain, and muscles, slow the heart rate so that the heart does not have to work so hard or need so much oxygen, prepare the lungs for breathing by dilating the bronchioles, cause fat and glycogen to be broken down and available for quick energy, and in all these ways prepare the baby for the demands of life outside the uterus.[47]

They also prompt you to release oxytocin, the hormone of contractions. "Oxytocin" means "fast birth," from the Greek "oxy," for fast, and "toc," for birth. Side effects of oxytocin include pain relief and a feeling of well-being. Synthetic oxytocin causes mighty contractions, but it does not have the same nice side effects as the real thing.

No matter how your labor starts or finishes, it will be an experience like no other. What kind of experience will be largely determined by God, fate, or nature, depending on your point of view. Still, your own desires and preparation can make a difference. Think about how you'd like to greet your baby. Here are a few ideas for a gentle Birth Day.

*Keep Things Quiet*
Hormones are chemicals designed to work in primitive environments, without the interference of your rational brain, without verbal instructions from birth "coaches," without the knowledge that comes from medical degrees, without blinking and beeping machines. The primary requirement for a safe and physiologically normal birth is not to disturb the flow of hormones. In the birthing room, the atmosphere should be dark, private, and quiet. The right conditions will suppress adrenaline and allow oxytocin to flow. You need oxytocin to give birth, to deliver the placenta safely,

to prevent excess bleeding, and to bond with your baby. The "hormone of love," oxytocin reaches its lifetime peak in mothers and babies in the hours after a natural birth. Oxytocin also stimulates milk letdown. Oxytocin is the all-powerful hormone of birth, nursing, and love. During this critical period, let it flow.

### Get Some Time Naked

State-of-the-art care for premature babies does not necessarily mean placing them in a heated glass box, or incubator. The best hospitals use "kangaroo care," which involves nothing more than keeping the tiny baby in naked skin contact with its mother. Caregivers invented kangaroo care to serve the needs of premature babies where access to technology is poor. It is now used all over the world. Unable to regulate their own breathing and body temperature, premature babies benefit hugely from touch and warmth. Kangaroo care supports brain development, promotes maternal bonding, improves oxygen saturation levels, regulates the baby's temperature, aids breast-feeding, reduces the baby's stress hormones, and improves the baby's alert rest and sleep. Bigger babies only minutes old will like it too. Hold your baby naked against your skin right away. Delay unnecessary procedures, such as bathing or weighing the baby. Let her smell you, look at you, and root for your nipple if she's ready.

### Skip the Bath

Newborns are not dirty. The thick white stuff on your baby is called vernix caseosa, and it's good for him. In the womb, vernix is a barrier against amniotic fluid. After birth, vernix is a moisturizer, protecting his delicate skin from the sudden exposure to air. It also contains immune factors, such as lysozyme, lactoferrin, and secretory leukocyte protease inhibitor, which kill common perinatal pathogens, including group B *Streptococcus*, *K. pneumoniae*, *Listeria monocytogenes*, *Candida albicans*, and *E. coli*.[48] If you bathe your baby, do so gently, without wiping off the valuable vernix. It will disappear on its own.

## Don't Cut the Cord

Don't cut the umbilical cord until it's white and flaccid, ideally after you deliver the placenta. While the cord pulses, placental blood supplies the baby's lungs, kidneys, liver, intestines, and skin—organs she is using for the first time—with oxygen, red blood cells, and immune and clotting factors. Leaving the cord intact is equivalent to giving the baby a blood transfusion at a sensitive time. A seven-pound baby has about 240 milliliters of blood in his body. Cutting the cord robs the baby, on average, of 100 milliliters of blood. Cord blood also contains nutrients such as zinc. Newborn iron levels are significantly higher when the cord remains intact.[49] Just before birth, the mother transfers brain-building choline and betaine to her baby. Cord blood contains much more of both than maternal blood.[50] Give your baby a Birth Day dose of real food.

## Give the Baby Some of Your Bacteria

If you have a cesarean, you will want to give your baby some bacteria. According to 2010 research by Dr. Maria Dominguez-Bello of the American Microbiome Institute, the biome of babies born vaginally matches the mother's birth canal (dominated by beneficial *Lactobacillus*) while babies born via surgery acquire colonies typical of the skin surface, populated by too much potential harmful *Staphylococcus*. Dominguez-Bello has tested swabbing the baby's mouth, nose, and skin with gauze inoculated for one hour in the mother's birth canal. At four months, the swabbed cesarean babies do show healthy vaginal bacteria.

Waiting for the Birth Day is exciting. But don't let it be nerve-wracking. In the ninth month, your chief goal is to feel calm. Concentrate on your own fitness—mental, physical, and spiritual—not on the calendar. Eat well, drink plenty of water, get lots of rest, and don't let anyone talk you into being induced without a first-rate reason. You're not submitting a tax return. You're having a baby.

## BIRTH DAY

On October 12, I was thirty-eight weeks pregnant and feeling grim about the state of modern obstetrics. I posted a little essay on my Web site.

> In the October 9, 2006, issue of the *New Yorker*, Atul Gawande ("The Score: How Childbirth Went Industrial") does a good job reciting the history of increasingly violent, and increasingly routine, interventions in the natural physiology of birth. Alas many of these (such as electronic fetal monitoring) increase cesarean rates. The cesarean is indeed a "magnificent rescue operation," as Michel Odent—a surgeon, obstetrician, and midwife—has called it, and in true emergencies we are grateful for it. But it's unfortunate that there is . . . a "genuine" debate about whether a healthy mother with no medical risk factors would choose a cesarean. The September 2006 issue of *Birth: Issues in Perinatal Care* reported on a study of nearly six million births. After adjusting for medical risks, socioeconomic factors, and common causes of neonatal death (such as congenital malformations), researchers found that babies born by cesarean section were twice as likely to die than babies born vaginally.

Later that day, Linda felt my belly and said, "I can't say for sure, but this baby might be breech." My heart sank. When you're nine months pregnant, you hope the baby is head down, the optimal position. The smooth, heavy head puts pressure on the cervix, which aids dilation and delivery. Breech means that either the baby's bottom or its feet are pointing down. About 3 to 4 percent of babies are breech at the end of pregnancy. Sometimes they turn at the last minute. Sometimes they don't.

I considered getting an ultrasound "for position only," which would mean taking a quick picture of the baby. Almost certainly harmless, I thought. So said Linda and other midwives I asked. For reasons I can't explain, I decided against it. The boys at the bike shop helped me inflate the birthing pool, a basic backyard number for kids I bought online. A bulbous blue thing covered in pink and yellow fish, it filled up all the floor space in the bedroom and looked ridiculous. Underneath the bed was a twenty-five-foot garden hose. I had no idea we would never touch the hose or fill the tub.

My mother came to visit. We went around town, going to the farmers' market and buying my first baby items; tiny T-shirts, lots of cloth diapers, a green potty. In week thirty-nine, Linda found the baby head down, spine against my belly. Just what you want. "Am relieved," says my diary. "Feel v ready anytime. Feel head clear." Forty weeks was four days away. I went for a walk-run on the treadmill and poached a chicken for Cobb salad. That night at the movies, I sat between Rob and my mother. After about thirty minutes, I poked Rob and pointed down. "Contractions." The pangs were stronger than the slight tugging feeling I'd had for about two weeks—"practice" contractions called Braxton Hicks, after the English doctor who identified them in 1872. Back at the apartment, I made us all a Cobb salad, had a glass of wine, and climbed into bed.

On October 23, I woke up with a backache and labored all day. By six o'clock every contraction hurt a lot. *Tonight*, I thought, *there's going to be a baby*. Linda examined me. To my surprise I hadn't dilated. I made myself some scrambled eggs, but I wasn't hungry. Rob brought me orchids and ice cream. When Linda examined me again later that evening, nothing had changed. "Have some ice cream and wine and go to sleep," she said as she left.

The wine and ice cream weren't palatable. Contractions were more painful than I ever imagined, like a chisel hammering my tailbone. All night they came. "Tell me I can do it!" I would roar, "TELL ME!" and then fall back to sleep, even for five minutes, before the next wave would creep up and crest with a punishing strike. Around one A.M., Linda came back and slept on the couch. In the morning, no news. Linda was calm and direct. "We need to go to the hospital," she said. Her meaning did not sink in.

## FOOD AND DRINK DURING LABOR

**In some hospitals, policy forbids laboring women to eat or drink, but you may suck ice chips. I suspect the main reason is to keep your stomach empty in case the doctor wants to give you drugs that cause nausea. It's a shame. A woman in labor should eat and drink as she pleases. Still, I was surprised to learn that not eating—even for many hours—is also perfectly normal. Many books counsel women in labor to eat. ("You need energy!") Yes, you do, but not necessarily from a banana. Giving birth and running a marathon are not alike. Unlike your legs, the uterus is made of smooth, or involuntary, muscle. It runs on fat, not glucose. The uterus works effectively without sugar. You may, however, want to turn off the neocortex, which runs on glucose. (That's why you feel lightheaded and stupid when blood sugar drops.) Oxytocin flows faster when the neocortex is down, not up, which means that, other things being equal, labor will go more smoothly if your brain is not alert from quick-energy carbohydrate.**

I had imagined an emergency, of course. But the emergency I had pictured involved (perhaps) bleeding, an oxygen mask, an ambulance, and the hospital just blocks away. It had not occurred to me that I might leave the apartment on my own two feet and ride in Linda's car to a maternity ward twenty-five miles away. Linda had other plans. When you've attended four hundred home births, you can see when babies need help. We were heading for her excellent backup hospital. It was the roughest ride of my life. I yelped all the way.

At the hospital, the chief midwife found me about two to three centimeters dilated and the baby LOP—left occipital posterior. That means the baby, who had started labor with its back toward my belly, was now lying with its spine to my spine, a position called "back labor." Back labor isn't easy. That would explain the hammering feeling, spine grating on spine, and lack of dilation. The question is what to do about posterior babies. Probably nothing. A large Australian study found that a common midwifery tactic—having the woman rock on her hands and knees from thirty-seven weeks until labor starts—did not reduce the number of posterior babies.[51] Even late in labor, most posterior babies—about 80 percent, says one study—turn to be born.[52]

For the next three hours, I labored in various positions the hospital midwife recommended. When I still hadn't dilated properly, she called for an epidural—a shot of painkillers to the spine. I was confused. The pain was intense, but I wasn't particularly looking for relief. I was looking for a baby. The logic of the epidural in a case like mine is this: You're exhausted from prolonged, unproductive back labor; with pain relief, you'll relax, dilate, and push the baby out, as the drugs wear off and sensation returns. That is indeed what allows some women to have a vaginal birth.

The epidural did its job. Below the waist, I was numb, as advertised. From my perspective both the contractions and pain were gone. In every other respect, I felt worse. A needle in my back delivered the drugs. A needle in my wrist gave me fluids. I wore a catheter. The electronic fetal monitor glued to a half-dozen spots on my body measured the baby's heart rate, my heart rate, and the contractions. Soon my legs were painfully swollen. Physically, I have never been more miserable.

That was not the most painful blow. After I was hooked up to the monitors, no one looked at me. Not the nurses, not the midwives. Not even my mother. They looked at the blinking lights, graphs, and numbers on the machines. The busy machines beeped noisily, graphing contractions I couldn't feel. I lay passive. There was nothing else to do.

Many American women know the feeling. In 2001, 54 percent of birthing women had an epidural.[53] The epidural has a number of effects. It slows and lengthens labor. It doubles the chances Pitocin—synthetic oxytocin—will be used to spur contractions, doubles the chances forceps will be used, doubles the risk of severe tearing, and increases the rate of cesarean sections.[54] Especially in first-time mothers.[55] In babies, epidural drugs cause reduced muscle tone, decreased sucking, lower neurobehavioral scores, and higher rates of jaundice.[56] The most comprehensive database on the long-term effects of using drugs in labor shows worrisome links to drug addiction in teens.[57]

Three hours later, my labor was still stalled. The hospital midwife gave me Pitocin, hoping to move things along with more powerful contractions. Time wore on. Now there was truly nothing to do. Contractions—not your own—come and go. Pitocin does it all for you. Except that Pitocin didn't work. About thirty-four hours after labor started, I had a cesarean section.

The moment I had hoped to avoid but never really pictured arrived. I was beyond tears. The anesthesiologist topped up the epidural with another cocktail of painkillers. I was wheeled into the operating room, where nurses strapped my arms down in case the the anesthesiologist needed ready access to my IV. A curtain separated my face from my belly.

It was October 24. My due date. There was some calm bustling—the efficient sounds of people going through familiar motions, not unlike the griddle cook in a busy diner. Being awake during major surgery is odd. You're the focus of concentration, yet ignored. About fifteen minutes later, there was a tugging. Someone said, "Almost there." Then a loud wail and quiet cheers. My forty weeks were over.

At my request, no one announced the baby's sex. I listened helplessly to my baby cry while the surgeon and nurses checked its vital signs. I kept calling out, "Hello, Little Baby!" The anesthesiologist unstrapped my left arm. After several long minutes, the surgeon—the baby-faced Dr. Andrew Garber, who both respects midwifery and knows when babies need to be rescued—stood above me, holding a blurry pink creature, arms and legs flapping. "Oh, Little Baby," I said, tears running down my face. "You're a *boy*."

## CHAPTER 4

# Nursing Your Baby

### VERY SOGGY INDEED

I cried every day for a month. Except on November 11, when my diary says, "Didn't cry today!" I guess I thought it was all behind me. But tears returned the next day, and the next. How much was hormones, how much joy, how much disappointment that I'd had a baby by surgery, how much gratitude that the baby—Julian Charles—was alive and well, no one can say.

What we can say is that it's a rare new mother who isn't tearful. The third day, apparently, produces a particularly strong cocktail of tear-jerking hormones. Crying is quite common and perfectly normal. Hormones are realigning themselves. You may be just a little tearful or wail away for weeks. Poignant things, like helpless animals or starving kids in distant countries, may set you off.

Proper depression is another story. If you're hopeless, apathetic, angry, grief-ridden, or unable to cope with the daily routine of baby care, you may have a case of postnatal depression, which requires immediate professional attention. Depressed mothers and their babies are at risk. Taking antidepressants—even while nursing—may be better for your baby than having a depressed mother.

Meanwhile, being well fed can prevent mild baby blues. Pregnancy may have sapped you, but you can recover while nursing. The best book on postnatal depression and food I've seen is *Rebuilding from Depression*, by Amanda Rose, who understands the condition from bitter experience. "The rich get richer and the poor get poorer," she writes. "We have at least three generations of nutritional poverty in my family . . . Grandmother bequeathed her vitamin and mineral stores to my mother who bequeathed an ever-dwindling supply to me. My grandmother did not even have the courtesy to pass on her movie star good looks as part of the package. But her body had no choice but to pass on a poor supply of B vitamins." Eat plenty of fish, red meat, liver, and whole grains for these brain boosters: omega-3 fats, iron, zinc, and B vitamins, especially $B_{12}$.

Along with weeping, count on some leaking. When my milk came in, Julian and I hadn't got the hang of nursing. Oh, we were nursing, if you call "nibbly-kissy-sucky" nursing. That's mostly what he was up to, according to my technically precise notes. Precious little milk went down his throat. Two days after the surgery, my breasts turned into watermelons. Leaky, squirting watermelons, bigger than his head, with way more milk than he could drink. For five days, they were painfully big and hard. When I tried to ease my discomfort by "expressing" milk, it shot across the shower a good fifteen inches, hitting the tiles with surprising force.

That's how I discovered that women have four or five holes in each nipple, not one. When you squeeze your breast, milk leaves the nipple from all these tiny exits, each stream pointing in a different direction, little milk-beams crossing like lights in the night sky. According to myth, the Milky Way was created when the demigod Hercules nursed from the goddess Hera, and her milk sprayed across the sky. This poetic tale is told in rich pinks and blues in Jacobo Tintoretto's sixteenth-century masterpiece, *The Origin of the Milky Way*.

When your breasts are engorged, expressing milk can ease short-term discomfort and help a newborn get hold of a breast that's too big and hard. But in the long run, it's counterproductive because the breasts, thinking you are a hungry baby, will respond to your signals and make more. Eventually, your milk supply will ease off to match your baby's appetite. Your breasts will be softer. Conversely, twins will cause your milk supply to rise. It's all determined by the amount and frequency of sucking. A true undersupply of milk is rare. The best approach is good nutrition and lots of nursing. Your milk will come. And it won't stop until the baby stops nursing.

Your breasts are not the only thing leaking. Newborns pee and poop frequently, and they do so round the clock. The good news is that baby pee is much like water, and breast-fed poop is as benign as bright yellow yogurt, in texture and scent. There will also be some spewing. Your baby may drink milk greedily and send it back without so much as a warning burp. You may be startled when this happens, but the baby usually recovers quickly. Unlike adults, newborns are often hungry shortly after spitting up. A few cycles of nursing and spitting up, even in the course of one evening, is nothing to worry about.

With all the dripping, leaking, and squirting, all those lovely baby things, and many others never intended for baby uses, will be saturated, soaked, sodden. Nightgowns, underpants, bras, diapers, blankets, sheets, and towels, not to mention chairs, couches, and rugs, need constant dabbing and mopping. Laundry is a daily affair. "It's a very soggy time period," writes Erica Lyon in *The Big Book of Birth*. "Very soggy indeed."

Someone else can do the laundry—and make dinner, too. Your chief activity is nursing. You'll easily find yourself in the nursing chair for eight hours a day. But once you and the baby figure it out, you can let your mind wander, read, talk on the phone, even doze. If you get lots of help with practical matters and gently surrender to your baby's needs, unpredictable as they seem, things will go more smoothly.

The soggy days found me dwelling on my labor and surgery. I read and reread my cesarean blog, written just twelve days before I had my very own: "The cesarean is indeed a 'magnificent rescue operation' . . . and in true emergencies we are grateful for it." Was I ever grateful. We needed help and we got it. But I couldn't stop crying. Driven to figure out why it happened, I pored over obstetrical journals and midwifery books.

The geometry of human birth is surprisingly precise. All being well, the narrowest bit of the typical fetal head can just pass through the widest part of the typical pelvis. When he cut me open, Dr. Garber found Julian in an extremely rare position called by the forbidding name "transverse arrest." A baby in transverse arrest presents the widest part of his head to the cervix and pelvis and gets stuck there. Even if the cervix dilates completely, the baby cannot pass the pelvic "spines," as the pointy bones on either side of the exit are known. The average fetal head is eleven centimeters from front to back. The pelvic spines are nine to ten centimeters apart. You see the problem.

One day I did see the problem—literally. The diagram of a baby's head lodged in the spines in *Understanding and Teaching Optimal Fetal Positioning* could not be clearer. It called to mind trying to get a picnic table through a door sideways. This drawing, easily worth its thousand words, was accompanied by a straightforward assessment neatly condensed to just five: "There is no way out."

This sentence made an impression. Midwifery books, if you aren't familiar with them, are brimming with gentle methods for turning babies in not-perfect positions in order to have a safe vaginal birth. Experienced midwives have great confidence with posterior, breech, and other oddly placed babies. So do certain pregnant women. The strength and conviction, often spiritual, of these mothers and midwives are notable.

After doing all my homework, it seemed to me that Julian and I had the right care. We had the benefit of spontaneous labor, and more than twenty-four hours of natural contractions. When we needed help, we got it. Transverse arrest is precisely the sort of rare situation that has justly earned the cesarean the sobriquet "magnificent rescue operation." Even the best midwifery maneuvers were probably incapable of dislodging Julian's lovely head. Most important, mother and baby were thriving.

But logic and analysis only got me so far. I still felt sorry for myself. Why me? Why was *my baby* the one in this rare position, the one in need of rescue? One day, my mother stopped the navel-gazing. She pretended to be Julian. "Thank you," she said, "for allowing me to be born in the way that was safest for me." Simple, brilliant, original—classic Susan Planck. That line, which I whispered over his head for days, broke the emotional logjam. Of course Julian was a gift. But from that moment on, I saw the surgery itself as another gift. I rewrote my story.

> A baby born at home grows up on a farm. She watches chickens lay eggs and cats give birth. She believes in a woman's ability to give birth. She dreams of having her own baby at home and quietly prepares. Publicly, she warns about the risks of cesareans. She has her baby by cesarean. She discovers firsthand what technology can do for mothers and babies and what it cannot. The woman is humbler. It is only the first lesson she will learn from her son.

In the first weeks, I often thought of Molly, the dancer I'd met that day at prenatal yoga. The soggy days are disorganized days, but I managed to dig out her phone number, and to my delight she called right back. The first question is standard. *How did the birth go?* I told my tale, including the surprise excursion into modern surgical birth, the self-pity, and the happy ending. She listened so sympathetically; I know I went on a bit.

At last she spoke. "You're not going to believe this." At once I knew, as you probably do, what she was about to say. As you may recall, Molly was the only woman I met in forty weeks who shared my hopes for a natural birth. She was also the only one who had her baby by cesarean. When I saw Molly and met her winsome son at a TriBeCa nursing circle not long after, they were doing great.

## PRO·LIFE

Probiotics—meaning "pro-life"—are the good bacteria in your body and in real food. They populate the gut, where they aid digestion, produce neurotransmitters, and boost immunity, among other tasks. Gut flora are astonishingly productive workers. They create energy by breaking down the food you eat. They produce vitamin $K_2$ and B vitamins. They keep the gut wall healthy. They train your immune system to identify and kill invaders. Many pathogens meet their maker in the gut before they make trouble in the rest of the body.

Though you can buy probiotics, the food business didn't invent these helpful little animals. The beneficial strains of *Bifidobacteria* and *Lactobacilli* occur naturally in raw milk, real yogurt, raw milk cheese, sauerkraut, and other traditional cultured and lacto-fermented foods. Probiotics contrast with antibiotics, which kill off pathogenic bacteria, and good ones, too. That's why you eat yogurt or take supplemental probiotics along with a course of antibiotics.

*Lactobacillus* and company are your friends. But these organisms are amateurs, mere bit players in health, compared with breast milk. When your baby is born, her immune system and digestive tract are immature. Breast milk doesn't merely give your baby's immune and digestive systems a helpful boost. It creates and finishes them.

In your womb, the baby's digestive tract is largely sterile. A trip down the birth canal begins to populate the baby's skin, ears, nose, throat, and gut with the right bacteria. As we've seen, cesarean babies miss out on this handy infiltration of good flora. But there is a backup plan. Your first milk, called colostrum, is a slightly thick, yellowish fluid which gathers in your breasts in late pregnancy. The rest of your milk doesn't come in until a few days after there's a baby to feed. Colostrum populates her gut with the right bacteria, including *Bifidus flora*. Even a small amount of formula, or any other foreign food, reshapes the bacterial village in the wrong fashion, so that within twenty-four hours it resembles the bacteria in an adult stomach, leaving your baby more vulnerable to infection.[1] Once the baby is back on breast milk, it takes two to four weeks to restore the right bacteria.

You don't find *Bifidus flora* in formula.

Some of the sugars in human milk, called oligosaccharides, are indigestible to the baby, but they are meat and drink to the good bacteria in her intestines. At least 130 known oligosaccharides, often called pre-biotics, take up residence in the gut, feeding the good guys. They also pass through it, heading for the respiratory tract, where they fight viral, bacterial, and protazoan parasite infections by preventing pathogens from binding to the baby's tissues.

You don't find oligosaccharides in formula. Or rather, when you do, they fail to have the same desirable effects—that is, they don't feed *Bifidus flora*. Researchers who figured this out said, "Human milk oligosaccharides remain one hundred and thirty reasons to breastfeed."[2]

Your baby's little colon is full of greenish or black sticky stuff called meconium. It doesn't move easily, but colostrum flushes it right out. If you nurse right away, your baby's first breast-milk poop—the yogurtlike stuff—will come within a few hours to two days.

Your milk doesn't merely fill your baby's stomach. It leaves a mark on it. Her intestine is porous and thus vulnerable to foreign bacteria and to antigens, proteins which might trigger allergies. Colostrum seals it up properly. Growth factors in your milk prompt your baby's intestinal mucosal lining to grow and develop. Your new baby cannot yet make enough of certain digestive agents, including amylase (the enzyme you need to digest starch) and bile salts, which digest fats. Breast milk provides both. Colostrum contains more amylase than mature milk.[3]

The newborn stomach is the size of a small marble. On the first day, it cannot stretch to accommodate more than about a half an ounce of milk. That's why babies fed with bottles can spit out the formula. They get too much. Your breast-fed baby will never overeat. It is impossible to force the breast on her.

The newborn immune system is another work in progress. Breast milk provides the finishing touch. The immunity provided by colostrum and mature milk beggars description. Dairy farmers know that newborn calves die without colostrum. Immune factors, including macrophages, leukocytes, IgG, and IgA, instantly and actively protect your newborn from countless new microbes she encounters. IgG and IgA are much more concentrated in colostrum than in mature milk, and they stimulate and enhance the immune system, preparing it for childhood and beyond. The most common whey proteins in your milk, lactalbumin and lactoferrin, also fight infections.

The immunity breast milk provides is tailored, reflecting the unique ecology you and your baby share. Within hours of encountering a pathogen, you produce antibodies which you pass to your baby through your milk. That's why it's natural for mothers to nuzzle, rub, kiss, and even lick their babies. You gather her germs with your mouth and skin, so that your breasts can make the antibodies she needs.

There are no antibodies in formula.

Those are merely the immediate protective effects of breast milk. Other agents prepare your baby's immune system for his entire life by promoting normal growth of the thymus, a gland devoted exclusively to immune function. Among other things, the thymus makes killer white blood cells called T cells. Loss of the thymus at an early age results in severe immunodeficiency and a high susceptibility to infection. Formula babies have abnormally small thymus glands, which may explain why they have more immune disorders than breast-fed babies.[4]

There are no immune factors to feed the thyroid in formula.

The American Academy of Pediatrics (AAP) recommends exclusive breast-feeding for six months and continuing to nurse for one year. "Exclusive" breast-feeding means no other food or liquid. The benefits of milk and nothing but for at least six months are substantial. In the first year of life, babies who drink artificial milk have a higher incidence of respiratory diseases such as pneumonia and bronchitis, diarrhea and other digestive illnesses, ear infections, urinary tract infections, and meningitis. They are more likely to be admitted to hospitals than nursing babies and to die suddenly, usually in bed (SIDS).[5] You can see why the World Health Organization calls colostrum the baby's "first immunization."

Infectious disease used to kill a lot of babies and children. That's why vaccines are a public health miracle. Widespread vaccination has nearly wiped out many diseases in the United States and Europe, and for this we're grateful. Still, some parents and doctors question the official vaccine schedule. We can't do justice to this complex topic here, so I'll simply note that my children are vaccinated, and make a pitch for breast-feeding. Colostrum and breast milk amount to a whole-body, multidisease, natural vaccine for your baby for as long as you nurse. In *The Vaccine Book: Making the Right Decision for Your Child*, Dr. Robert Sears covers the debate. Neither for vaccines nor against them, Sears is for choice. What he says about breast milk, however, is unequivocal.

> Breast milk has antibodies that coat the lining of the nose, lungs, and intestines, so most germs that get inhaled or swallowed are killed. When I see patients . . . who tell me they don't want their baby to get vaccines, my first response is, "I hope you plan to breast-feed your baby for at least two years!" If the parents answer, "Yes, of course we are," I breathe a sigh of relief. Breast milk passes a whole host of mom's antibodies for a variety of diseases to the baby. If they tell me, "Well, no. We just weaned our two-month-old and are now using formula," I worry. Of course, even a breastfed baby can get sick. But the chances are lower . . . Furthermore, if an unvaccinated baby is in day care *and* is not breast-fed, he is really asking to get sick. Parents who choose not to vaccinate should avoid day care and should breast-feed for as long as possible. It

would be prudent to avoid even church nurseries and health club childcare for the first year or two.

Breast-fed babies also have extra protection against arthritis, asthma, allergy, eczema, immune system cancers such as lymphoma, Crohn's disease, colitis, Hodgkin's disease, breast cancer, obesity, diabetes, stroke, and heart disease. Breast milk may prevent obesity and diabetes because it contains the protein adiponectin, which lowers blood sugar. Low adiponectin is linked to obesity, Type 2 diabetes, insulin resistance, and heart disease. Babies with digestive disorders such as cystic fibrosis and celiac disease do much better on breast milk than formula. Breast milk protects teeth by depositing phosphorus and calcium on enamel. Nursing mothers are protected against bladder infections, hip fractures, osteoporosis, Type 2 diabetes, and cancer of the breast, cervix, and ovary. Pregnancy is a metabolic challenge. When you breast-feed during what experts call the fourth trimester, it appears to reset your system.

Breast milk, in other words, is more than merely food. Most foods we can take or leave. If you don't happen to eat apples or beef, olive oil or scallops, there is a decent substitute for each nutrient you'll be missing. Yet every baby is designed to drink his mother's milk. There are many imitations, but there is no substitute. Like nothing else we call food, breast milk is pro-life.

## YOUR MILK AND YOUR DIET

Your milk is all your baby needs until he is six months old. If you're reasonably well fed, your milk will contain just the right amount of protein, fat, carbohydrate, and all the other nutrients his body wants. He doesn't need cereal, sweet potatoes, banana, meat, or even a sip of water. He doesn't need vitamins, minerals, or fiber. Breast milk is a complete meal. I find this amazing.

You have your hands full with a newborn. It's no small relief that you don't have to think about your baby's diet. The recipe for breast milk is time-honored and—conveniently for you—automatic. Consider vitamin C. Most mammals can make it, but not humans. We have to get it from food, and babies have to get it from breast milk. Thirty minutes after you eat an orange, vitamin C appears in your milk, just like that.

The nursing diet is simple. Just keep eating the same good foods you ate in the last forty weeks. Many nursing women are hungry and thirsty. The people of Papua New Guinea believe fish soup and coconut water support milk production. It's no surprise that many traditional postpartum foods, like chicken soup, are liquids. Water is important when you're nursing. The pregnancy exercise expert James Clapp found that nursing women who exercise automatically eat more to compensate for the extra calories they're burning—about five hundred calories daily at four months—but they do not spontaneously drink more water. All this means is that you may need to remind yourself to refill your glass. If your pee is yellow, you're not drinking enough.

Specific foods for increasing milk supply have a long history in folk medicine, but I've found little compelling evidence for them. Oatmeal is probably the most famous lactogenic food; I still don't know why. In Peru and Africa, Weston Price found nursing women eating special soaked grains, particularly red millet and quinoa. They were significantly richer in calcium than other grains. Fine. But as a source of calcium, grains are probably second-best to milk, chicken soup, and small fish with bones.

Not so long ago, American doctors told nursing mothers to drink stout, and in Germany and the Dominican Republic, they drink low-alcohol malt beer. According to Dr. Thomas Hale, author of the definitive *Medications and Mother's Milk*, a polysaccharide from barley in alcoholic and nonalcoholic beer alike stimulates prolactin, the main nursing hormone. Perhaps it works.

My theory, unproven, about porridge, beer, and nursing, goes like this: A poor or malnourished woman—say, during the

Irish potato famine or the droughts that strike farming tribes—
lacks adequate animal foods. She survives on carbohydrates,
such as oats, potatoes, and millet, while the nutrient-dense foods,
such as beef and butter, are tightly rationed. Perhaps she spares
them for the working men and teenagers in her family. She needs
carbohydrates to keep weight on, and she needs to stay hydrated.
Beer is an inexpensive, liquid carbohydrate. It doesn't spoil and
may be more sterile than the local drinking water. If her diet is
poor, minute quantities of vitamin $B_{12}$ in fermented beer may
stave off deficiency. In short, I suspect that a bowl of oats and a
beer are the poor man's remedy for nourishing his nursing wife.
Good in a pinch, but what she needs is a steak.

What about a glass of wine? The studies on alcohol and nursing are incomplete. We don't know how much alcohol reaches
breast milk and what dose is harmful. It's said to disrupt sleep in
babies. Nevertheless, the data suggest that light to moderate drinking is safe for nursing babies. The American Academy of Pediatrics, La Leche League, and Dr. Thomas Hale consider moderate
alcohol consumption compatible with nursing. Once you metabolize alcohol, it disappears from your milk. Hale suggests waiting a
few hours after drinking to nurse, but I confess that I didn't.

In natural-food and breast-feeding circles, one hears a lot
about steering clear of wheat, milk, citrus, nuts, and other foods
to avoid contaminating breast milk. Although I know mothers
who swear that eliminating one food or another did a world of
good, I suspect these worries are overblown. Don't go crazy trying to pinpoint the cause and effect between, say, having a piece
of whole wheat toast (or peanut butter or cow milk) and your
baby's crying, sleeping heavily, waking frequently, diarrhea, or
constipation. A few babies react to foods their mothers eat. For
most healthy nursing pairs, special diets are seldom necessary.
The pediatrician Michel Cohen agrees:

> I've seen many mothers confine themselves to a stringent diet,
> with one result: unhappiness. First theirs, then the baby's.

And I've seen thousands of other mothers who ate whatever they felt like, just as they did before they were pregnant, without any problem. For the benefit of everyone around you, don't deprive yourself. Enjoy varied meals, and maintain a good diet. Don't think in terms of specific nutrients, like protein, iron, calcium, or fluoride. They're all included in well-rounded meals.

I did find one interesting link between breast milk, eczema, and allergies. The merrier the mother, the less eczema and the fewer allergies to dust mites and latex in the baby.[6] How does that work? People with eczema tend to have less melatonin. When a nursing mother laughs, melatonin levels in her milk rise. In this study, the laughing mothers watched Charlie Chaplin in the film *Modern Times* while the others got the weather report. (No one said participating in clinical research was fair.)

Breast milk *will* taste different, from day to day, compared with the fixed "flavor profile" in formula. According to the Monell Chemical Senses Center, flavors from your diet, including garlic, pass to your milk. (Garlic can even be detected in amniotic fluid, which the baby drinks.) The changing flavor of your milk is probably good. Perhaps it will contribute to a more adventurous palate; we don't know. It does not mean that your milk tastes "funny" or that your baby can't digest it. In one study, babies preferred to nurse when the mother had garlic first.[7] Advice to avoid strong or spicy foods is unfounded.

Babies love breast milk. Apart from the fabulous container, what's the attraction? For one thing, it's sweet. Human milk is noticeably thinner and sweeter than cow milk. Breast milk is also a savory food. According to a 2000 study in the *Journal of the American College of Nutrition*, human milk contains the free (unbound) form of the amino acid glutamic acid. Researchers found that human milk contains five times more free amino acids than soy and milk formulas. Free glutamic acid is found in every food containing protein. It is responsible for one of the basic human tastes: *umami*, a Japanese word meaning some-thing like "pleasant savory taste." Free glutamic acid (the only kind you can taste) is found in a variety of popular foods, in-cluding beef, chicken, turkey, meat broths, fish, Parmigiano Reggiano, mushrooms, tomatoes, and fermented and aged foods, such as soy and fish sauce. As the makers of synthetic glutamic acid (monosodium glutamate) well know, this amino acid is also a flavor-enhancer. The *umami* boost accounts for classical reci-pes, such as Japanese broth, which begins with kombu and bo-nito flakes, or the Italian trio of tomato sauce, mushrooms, and Parmigiano Reggiano.

When Julian was nine months old, a pediatrician told me that breast milk doesn't contain enough vitamin D to prevent rickets. The American Academy of Pediatrics (AAP) recom-mends that every breast-fed baby take supplemental vitamin D for one year, or until she drinks one pint of vitamin D–fortified milk daily.[8] In 2010, the AAP said that formula-fed babies should take supplements too.

At first, the problem seems odd. How good can breast milk be if it can't prevent rickets? Why would human milk lack vita-min D, which is essential for strong bones and teeth? Babies sprout teeth from tooth buds created *in utero* in the first six months. In the first year, the skeleton grows fast. Yet most babies in the world are dependent on breast milk for six months to one year, as babies have always been. I wondered about the AAP policy, and of course I wondered whether Julian was getting enough vitamin D, so I looked into the matter.

Nutrition politics makes strange bedfellows. When I asked traditional food advocates about the AAP guidance, the an-swer was swift and stern. "Of course, breast milk is deficient in vitamin D. Women eating refined foods don't get enough vitamin D."

What is the answer here?

The AAP has a point. Vitamin D deficiency—and even rickets—is coming back. It's clear that some people with dark skin and some who live in northern climes do not get enough sun, especially in the winter, to produce enough vitamin D from cholesterol. The real-food people are also right about our sad industrial diet. Traditional diets contained ten times more vitamin D than modern ones. But it's quite different to conclude, first, that the breast milk of every woman is deficient and, second, that every breast-fed baby needs supplements. I'm not sure this is true, and I think it may needlessly worry nursing mothers. The mammary gland does raid the body for nutrients the baby needs, and what vitamin D breast milk contains is highly absorbable.

If you get some sun and eat real food, you probably don't need to worry about whether your nursing baby gets enough vitamin D. It's perfectly safe for you and your baby to walk or sit in the sun for a spell each day, although it's impossible to say how much vitamin D you'll make. The more skin you reveal, the better. As for dinner, crab, herring, pork, and cod liver oil are good sources of vitamin D. One study found that taking cod liver oil is better at raising vitamin D levels in breast milk than simply changing diet alone.[9]

Julian did not take synthetic vitamin D, as the doctor recommended. Nor did I. We did—and do—eat foods rich in vitamin D. From seven months to one year, Julian sampled—and actually ate—plenty of seafood, pork, and dairy. He did not drink a pint of milk fortified with vitamin D daily. He didn't much care for cow milk until much later. We don't buy fortified milk; we drink whole milk with its natural vitamins. At about one year, Julian began taking cod liver oil. The summer he was five months old, he went outdoors naked, without sunscreen. That summer, he got some sun every day—even on his bottom. So did I.

The single most important ingredient in your milk is fat. About 50 percent of the calories in breast milk come from fat. Your baby needs fat for weight gain and energy. She needs fat to assimilate protein, calcium, and fat-soluble vitamins. Your baby depends on enzymes in your milk, such as lipase, to digest fat.

Her pancreas won't make enough lipase for four to six months, but when she's only a week old, your baby absorbs 90 percent of the fat in your milk.[10] That's how good mother's milk is.

Unfortunately, fats attract and store fat-soluble poisons. There is ample evidence of dangerous chemicals in breast milk, including three of the most famous persistent organic pollutants (POPs) in environmental toxicology: dioxins, DDT (still lingering, although it was banned in 1972), and polychlorinated biphenyls (PCBs). Thanks to biomagnification, a nursing baby consumes many times more POPs than his mother by weight, and the longer a baby nurses, the more chemicals he consumes. Researchers can trace POPs in twenty-five-year-olds to their mother's milk.

When I learned all this, I was shocked. I was thirty-five years old, and it was the first bad thing I'd ever heard about breast milk. Mothers need to know whether breast milk is still best. Yes, it is. Recent studies favor breast milk, however polluted, over artificial milk.[11] A study of Dutch toddlers found no negative effects from chemicals in breast milk. Prenatal exposure to PCBs did prove harmful, however. Another Dutch study confirmed both conclusions: Prenatal chemicals are dangerous, and the benefits of breast milk outweigh the risks. An authoritative study of Michigan children found that PCBs in cord blood depressed IQ scores, while above-average levels of PCBs in milk did not.

As in adults, each kind of fat in mother's milk plays an important role in your baby's health. Monounsaturated fats are anti-inflammatory and good for immunity. Saturated fats help assimilate omega-3 fats and lay down calcium. Mother's milk is a rare source of the saturated fat lauric acid. Antimicrobial and antiviral, lauric acid is so critical to the baby's immunity that it must, by law, be added to infant formula. The usual source is coconut oil. Lauric acid and other fats in your milk— good and bad—are directly related to what you eat. A spoonful of virgin coconut oil daily is a great food for nursing mothers. As

## NUTRIENTS IN (MY) BREAST MILK

|  | NUMBER OF GRAMS (PER 100G MILK) |
|---|---|
| **Total Fat** | 2.52 |
| **Saturated fat** | 1.39 (55%) |
| **Monounsaturated fat** | 0.67 (27%) |
| **Polyunsaturated fat** | 0.46 (18%) |
| **Trans fat** | 0 |
| **Lactose** | 2.90 |
| **Protein** | 1.39 |

SOURCE: N. Planck milk, November 20, 2006 (Analysis by Intertek.)

we'll see shortly, polyunsaturated fats are indispensable for eye and brain development.

Curious about the nutrients in my milk, I had it tested by a lab that writes official nutrition labels. (Today you can buy home testing kits.) Alas, the sample was too small to check all the vitamins. (I was hoping to prove the doctor wrong about vitamin D.) My milk, like all human milk, was fairly sweet, with more lactose than protein. It was about 2.5 percent fat, thin compared to whole Jersey cow milk, which is 4 to 6 percent fat. More than half of the fat is saturated. I find it odd that we're told to limit the natural saturated fats our babies eat.

One fat I absolutely did not want to find in my milk: trans fat. I'm pretty careful to avoid it, but you never know what's in restaurant food, and I was relieved to see none. Actually, the report said that trans fats in my milk were less than 0.05 percent of total fat. Because that comes to less than one half a gram for each one-hundred-gram serving, I could have printed NO TRANS

FATS on the label if I were to bottle and sell my milk in the dairy case at Murray's Cheese.

Trans fats in your milk enter the baby's tissues, where they disrupt fat metabolism, disable prostaglandins, and cause atherogenesis, all of which contribute to obesity, diabetes, and heart disease. The more trans fat you eat during pregnancy and nursing, the more trans fat in your milk. One study found that German breast milk contained 4.5 percent trans fats—less than American breast milk, but more than African breast milk, as trans fat consumption in each country would predict.[13] Other studies find that trans fats make up 2 to 18 percent of human milk.[14] That would displace a lot of good fats the baby needs.

Here's a striking fact. Once trans fat and fat-soluble pesticides (POPs) are in your body, the most efficient way to decontaminate your body of these fat-soluble poisons is to nurse your baby. The faster you lose weight while nursing, the more trans fat in your milk and the more trans fat the baby drinks. When you stop eating pesticides and trans fat, your fat will be cleaner. As you continue to nurse, your baby will drink cleaner milk. So will your next baby.

Every time I look at the research on pesticides and trans fats, I feel gloomy about industrial food all over again. Fortunately, it's getting easier to buy organic food and to avoid trans fat. Don't eat foods containing hydrogenated vegetable oils, including margarine, vegetable shortening, and cheap fried foods. Don't be confused about natural trans fat in grass-fed meat and butter. According to research by Flora Wang at the University of Alberta, trans vaccenic acid (VA), a naturally occurring trans fat, is good for you. The label won't tell you this. Sadly, the FDA hasn't noticed—or doesn't care—about the difference between humanmade and natural trans fats.

Mothers simply cannot escape the importance of fats. If only more doctors could help us choose good foods to feed our babies. In my dream pediatric practice, every pregnant and nursing mother would get a handout on fats. It would be very simple.

## DOCTOR'S ORDERS

### TRY NOT TO

- **Use or consume pesticides and other fat-soluble chemicals.**

### PLEASE DON'T

- **Eat trans fats when you're trying to conceive, pregnant, or nursing.**

### BE SURE TO

- **Eat a diverse diet of whole foods, including traditional fats.**
- **Eat clean wild fish or take fish oil while pregnant and nursing.**
- **Eat extra coconut, coconut milk, and coconut oil while nursing.**

### . . . AND DON'T HESITATE TO

- **Take cod liver oil and eat extra grass-fed butter if you think your diet isn't good enough.**

## THE QUEEN OF FATS

When Julian was about two weeks old, I squeezed some breast milk into a glass and tasted it. It was watery and sweet. It lacked the velvety texture of good cow milk—and the flavor, too, I thought. When I let it sit awhile, the cream rose to the top. It was sorry-looking, a thin yellow layer atop bluish milk, nothing like the satisfying inch or two of ivory cream from, say, a healthy Brown Swiss cow.

Still, I knew that little creamy layer was a precious commodity. I froze the milk, thinking Julian might drink it with a babysitter one day. He never did drink breast milk from a cup or bottle. More than a year later, I found the lonely milk in the freezer and sent it away, along with a fresh sample, to be tested for DHA, the Queen of Fats. The good DHA does for nursing babies is something to behold.

Remember the growth spurt fueled by fish in the third trimester? Here it comes again. In the first year, your baby's brain grows like mad. Delaying brain growth is the only way she can get out alive. The basic strategy of the human fetus is to hold the brain growth to the size of your pelvis, get out smoothly, and nurse furiously for a year or more.

Brain-wise, we are not like other mammals. At birth, the monkey brain is more than 65 percent of the size it will be in adulthood, but your baby's brain is only 25 percent of its full-grown size. Your baby is physically helpless. She won't be trotting after you any time soon, like a foal. She puts energy into her big brain, not her muscle. She's also somewhat hampered mentally, but that's no license to treat her like an idiot. It merely means her immature brain has a huge amount of growing to do before she pulls off fancy acts like speech.

Rapid brain growth is why they call the first three months of the baby's life the fourth trimester. Your newborn needs you

## OMEGA-3 FATS IN BREAST MILK

| BREAST MILK | OMEGA-6 TO OMEGA-3 RATIO |
| --- | --- |
| Canada (Inuit) | 3.8 |
| China (coastal) | 7 |
| Japan | 9.9 |
| China (urban) | 24 |
| China (rural) | 28 |
| United States* | 67 |
| United States* | 175 |

*Two studies

SOURCE: Andrew Stoll, *The Omega-3 Connection*

to keep eating brain food. Abundant research shows that more of these fats in your milk give nursing babies better intellectual, visual, and motor skills. For example, when mothers take cod liver oil during pregnancy and the fourth trimester, breast-fed babies score higher on intelligence tests at four years than the babies of mothers who consume corn oil.[15]

The fatty acids ARA and DHA are present in roughly equal amounts in the brain. Together they are essential for healthy brain development. It is not difficult to get ARA into your milk for your baby. ARA is found in meat, milk, and eggs, and you can make some, too. Most omnivores get plenty. You may want to pay more attention to getting enough DHA, which is found only in fish. The amounts of DHA in your diet, your milk, and your baby's blood rise and fall together.[16] A nursing mother who eats fish has ten times more DHA in her milk than one who doesn't.[17] Even cod liver oil, a relatively modest source of DHA and its precursor EPA, makes a difference. The breast milk of Norwegian women who take cod liver oil has higher levels of DHA.[18]

Traditional diets rich in fish contain significantly more omega-3 fat and less omega-6 fat than the typical American diet. As the table below shows, these fats duly show up in breast

## PERCENTAGE OF DHA IN BREAST MILK

| | |
|---|---|
| **Africa** | **0.07** |
| **Vegan** | **0.10** |
| **Canada, United States, Europe, Australia** | **0.20–0.30** |
| **Desirable** | **0.35** |
| **Japan** | **1.0** |

SOURCE: S. M. Innis, "Human Milk: Maternal Dietary Lipids and Infant Development," *Proceedings of the Nutrition Society* 66 (2007): 399.

milk. I've mentioned that an excess of omega-6 fats or a deficiency of omega-3 fats leads to obesity, diabetes, heart disease, and cancer. Most breast milk already meets and exceeds the baby's requirements for the omega-6 fat LA.[19] Whether you're nursing or not, the rule is simple: Eat more pink oil (salmon) and less yellow oil (corn).

As you can see from the table on page 153, the amount of DHA in breast milk varies widely. On average, Japanese breast milk contains ten times more DHA than vegan breast milk and fourteen times more DHA than African breast milk. It's not yet clear how much DHA is optimal in breast milk, only that deficiency is bad for the baby's eyes and brain. The evidence we have suggests that when the DHA drops below 0.35 percent of total fat, the baby's prospects are worse.[20] DHA made up 1.86 percent of the fats in my milk when Julian was three weeks old.[21]

Suppose it's your goal to make 0.35 percent of the fat in your breast milk DHA. How much fish do you need to eat? Unfortunately, we don't know that yet, either. The figures in the table below suggest that nursing mothers should consume more

## DHA IN MOTHER'S DIET AND BREAST MILK

|  | DHA IN MOTHER'S DIET (MG PER DAY) | DHA IN BREAST MILK (% OF TOTAL FAT) |
| --- | --- | --- |
| Canada* | 81 | 0.17 |
| Canada* | 131 | 0.34 |
| Desirable | Unknown | 0.35 |
| Norway | 200 | 0.50 |

*Two studies

SOURCE: S. M. Innis, "Human Milk: Maternal Dietary Lipids and Infant Development," *Proceedings of the Nutrition Society* 66 (2007): 399.

than 130 milligrams of DHA daily. We do know that fish oil is quite safe in large doses. Studies of pregnant women used 3,500 milligrams of EPA and DHA. Traditional diets contain much more. Eskimo women eating fish and seal may consume 14,000 grams of EPA and DHA daily. I took 1,000 to 3,000 milligrams of fish oil, plus extra cod liver oil, while pregnant and nursing. I've no idea how much DHA that represents, or how many omega-3 fats I get from the wild fish, grass-fed milk and beef, and pastured eggs I eat. Fish oil usually includes EPA, DHA, and other omega-3 fats, so if you're looking for DHA in particular, read the label.

When you nurse, the baby uses up your DHA. DHA loss is detectable after two months of nursing and usually levels off in a year. I tested my milk when Julian was three weeks old and again at sixteen months. During that period, the DHA in my milk fell from 1.86 percent to 1.4 percent of total fats, a decline of about 25 percent, even though I didn't change my diet. Clearly, Julian was draining DHA stores, but 1.4 percent was still well above the desirable level.

Sixty to 80 percent of the fat in your milk comes from your fat, not your lunch. That's probably because omega-3 fats at most times in human history were relatively rare and precious—you had to live near water to get any—and the infant's needs are immediate and huge. The baby "prefers" to take DHA from his mother's supply rather than rely on her uncertain diet.

Mothers keep EPA and DHA in a special place, known as gluteofemoral depots—in plain language, your bottom and thighs. Perhaps you've noticed that your body is rather protective of this fat. Even when you cut calories and lose weight, gluteofemoral fat is hard to move. *Except* during the third and the fourth trimesters—not by chance, the period of maximum brain growth. At this point, fat on your hips, thighs, and bottom is "selectively mobilized." Nice! This conjures up troops of fat cells marching off into the sunset. If you want to move fat, nurse your baby.

The fact that you're packing DHA in your hips has led to interesting speculation about mating behavior. It seems that men find women with thin waists and wide hips—that is, curves—more attractive than women with thick waists or no hips or both. The male preference for a low waist-to-hip ratio is widespread and consistent, from the United States to Europe, Japan, Uganda, Ecuador, and Kenya. In fifty-eight cultures, men prefer a low ratio 90 percent of the time. The waist-hip ratio even trumps whether the woman is fat or thin. Curves count.

Experts have surmised that curves signal fertility or general health, but the evidence is uneven. In 2008, an article in *Evolution and Human Behavior* presented a new and intriguing theory. Curvy women have smarter babies.[22] Men "know" this, and they want curvy women to bear their children.

The evidence for this startling hypothesis is equally startling. Curvy women are smarter, even after accounting for age, family income, race, and ethnicity. Their babies are smarter, too, even after accounting for family income and the intelligence of mother and father. First babies are smarter than second babies, which suggests maternal depletion of omega-3 fats. Singletons have cognitive advantages over twins, presumably because they have to share omega-3 supplies. A teen mother, who is still growing herself, competes with her own baby for omega-3 fats. Is that one reason the babies of teenagers are mentally impaired compared with babies of grown women? When the young mother is curvy, the negative effects in babies disappear.

The alert reader will notice that I find the research on fish oil and babies compelling. I'm pretty keen on fish for mothers. If you agree, keep eating clean, wild fish as you nurse your baby. If you don't eat fish, make a special effort to eat pastured egg yolks. If you can't find pastured eggs, "enriched" eggs are next best. A small study found that eating two omega 3-enhanced eggs daily for six weeks nearly doubled the percentage of DHA in mother's milk.[23] (You can tell your cardiologist that cholesterol and triglycerides were unchanged after eating fourteen eggs a week for six weeks.) Vegetarians who consume dairy may get small amounts of omega-3 fats from grass-fed milk and butter.

Unfortunately, there is no natural DHA in a vegan diet. The best plant sources of omega-3 fats are flaxseed oil and walnuts. Both are rich in an omega-3 fat called alpha-linolenic acid (ALA), which the body can convert to EPA and then to DHA. However, only 1 percent of ALA turns into EPA, and less than 0.1 percent becomes DHA.[24] "Although the conversion of ALA to DHA appears to be higher in women than in men, and increased in pregnancy, increased dietary intakes of ALA do not increase DHA in blood lipids of either pregnant women or their newborn infants," writes Sheila Innis, an expert on breast milk fats at the Child and Family Research Institute.[25]

We know that DHA in mother's milk is directly related to DHA in her diet. The breast milk of vegan mothers has half the DHA of nonvegetarian mother's milk.[26] Another study found the breast milk of women who eat fish has ten times more DHA than the breast milk of vegans.[27] Blood levels of DHA in babies of vegan mothers are less than one third of the blood levels in babies of omnivores.[28] Supplemental ALA does not affect breast milk levels of DHA, but eating foods containing DHA does raise DHA in breast milk and the baby's blood.[29]

I've considered the thorny issue of vegan diets for many years now. When I gradually gave up being a vegan, the first animal products I began to eat were eggs, yogurt, and fish. You can get the nutrients in eggs and milk elsewhere, but there's no good substitute for seafood in the human diet. Still, many dedicated vegetarians will choose never to eat fish, so I studied the research again. Can you be in good health without fish? I think you can. You can get what you need from real milk, yogurt, cheese, butter, and eggs.

Then I got pregnant. This time, I looked at the specific needs of mother and baby, and I looked closely. In this unique period of growth and development, I cannot see the sense in doing without dietary DHA. Nor would I settle for synthetic DHA and ARA created from algae and fungus. I can speak only for myself, but I wouldn't dream of nursing a little *Homo sapiens* without eating plenty of real fish. Nature made me an omnivore, and nature has her reasons.

## HARDER THAN IT LOOKS

Of all the sorry attempts to imitate traditional foods, the story of trying to mimic breast milk is the most disturbing. Until quite recently, we had little idea what was in breast milk or why babies needed it. In the preindustrial, Western world, 95 percent of babies were breast-fed by their mothers or wet nurses. The unlucky ones were "hand-fed" a mixture called pap. It was made of water or milk boiled with flour.[30] Most of these babies "failed to thrive," and no wonder. Never mind the immune factors and other unique properties of breast milk they were missing. With a diet so poor, pap babies were lucky to be weaned to solid foods, as many were, between seven months and a year. Eggs, meat, fish—any real food is vitally important to a baby fed only milk and flour.

Efforts to give hand-fed babies a better chance, often championed by advocates for the poor, began in earnest in the nineteenth century, when a number of formulas were patented.[31] In 1867, the German chemist Justus von Liebig, a pioneer in the "New Newtrition"—a revolution in thinking, the ancestor of nutritionism, which said that all foods could be reduced to fat, protein, and carbohydrate—introduced his "Soluble Food for Babies" in Europe, and soon it came to the United States. Liebig's formula, a mix of wheat flour, cow milk, malt flour, and potassium bicarbonate, was sold as a liquid and powder. His formula became famous and spawned many competitors.

By the 1890s, marketing artificial milk to middle-class mothers—including the practice of sending free samples by mail—was widespread. Some doctors even said that formula was superior to breast milk from wet nurses. Artificial feeding was considered scientific and modern. Less affluent mothers, both rural and urban, who did not buy commercial formula often made it at home from whole milk or "top" milk—the creamy part—because the higher butterfat content made it more digestible than the tough curds that form when skim milk is heated.

Improvements in these early, primitive formulas came fairly rapidly. The safety of water and cow milk, both major ingredients in baby formula, was critically important. Many hand-fed babies died simply for lack of sanitation. In the early twentieth century, reformers won improvements in general sanitation, including garbage disposal and water treatment. They campaigned for better dairy hygiene and milk handling in overcrowded, dirty, and often urban dairies. Many state and local authorities responded by imposing mandatory pasteurization of milk.

## BREAST IS BEST

Cow milk is a great food for older infants and young children, but it's easy to see why human milk is better for little babies. A few examples will do. Cow milk contains more protein than human milk and less whey, which makes cow milk harder for your baby to digest than breast milk. The main amino acid in human milk is cysteine, whereas the main one in cow milk is methionine, which the newborn liver cannot metabolize properly. The amino acid taurine, which is essential for nervous development, is abundant in breast milk and absent in cow milk. Human milk is sweeter than cow milk because it contains more lactose, which breaks down into glucose and galactose, which feed your baby's brain. Breast milk contains more cholesterol than cow milk. Cholesterol is essential to the baby's developing brain and nervous system. Breast milk supplies a baby with much more cholesterol than the average adult consumes, and it contains a special enzyme to ensure the baby absorbs the cholesterol fully. Cow milk contains more iron than human milk, yet babies absorb five times more iron from breast milk (nearly 50 percent) than from cow milk (10 percent).[32]

Heating milk was a mixed blessing. Certainly pasteurization prevented the spread of some diseases, such as brucellosis and tuberculosis, which were rampant in urban dairies, where cows were fed acidic pulp from nearby distilleries, and milking workers were often themselves contagious. But mandatory pasteurization, which came to New York City dairies in 1912 and many other American cities thereafter, also damages important heat-sensitive fats, vitamins, bacteria, and enzymes.

Still, better health through hygiene and nutrition seemed at hand. The home icebox made storage of milk or formula safe and convenient. By the 1920s, the practice of giving babies and children cod liver oil and orange juice had greatly reduced rickets and scurvy. Evaporated milk further decreased contamination in formulas.

These improvements—and they are no doubt improvements, in cleanliness and nutrition—had an unfortunate effect. From the 1930s to the 1960s, breast-feeding declined steadily. White, wealthy, urban, and educated mothers set the trend.[33] Early introduction to solid foods was also in vogue. Mothers fed their babies cow milk and cereals earlier and earlier, as early as four months.

You can picture all this, thanks to the bossy, kindhearted Aunt Belle. "Her niece, Mary, found Aunt Belle's letters about babies so very helpful that they have been made into a book for the use of other mothers who need simple help in the nursery," begins the preface to *Aunt Belle's Baby Book*, published in 1921 by the Mennen Company, makers of talcum powder and other baby products in Newark, New Jersey. Belle is the sort of aunt every new mother should have. "Aunt Belle has made the study of babies her life-work," it says. "Aunt Belle loves babies so much that she is always delighted to receive letters from their mothers, telling about them and their little problems."

As one would expect, Aunt Belle urges her readers to use Mennen soap and talcum powder, but the fact that *Aunt Belle's Baby Book* is a vintage example of advertorial is not my point. In eleven letters addressed to her niece, a young mother of twins, this slim handbook represents state-of-the-art baby care—also known as "scientific mothering"—for a middle-class household in 1921.

Mary's darling twins, Jack and Polly, were a surprise. (No ultrasound.) First, Aunt Belle advised finding arsenic-free paint for the nursery. She assumed that cloth diapers were hand-made, as were baby clothes made of cashmere, wool, silk, and cotton. The babies were to be breast-fed. ("Mother's milk is the one perfect food for babies.") They must be fed on a strict schedule, every three hours up to six P.M., then at ten P.M. and two A.M. "Being absolutely regular as to meal time is essential," wrote Aunt Belle. "Very soon they will wake themselves like little alarm-clocks."

Aunt Belle declared it "no wonder" that Mary hadn't enough milk for two babies, so they should also get a bottle. Aunt Belle was pleased that the formula Mary used was just like the one at the hospital where she worked: whole raw milk, boiled water, and malt or cane sugar. Belle was very strict about the cleanliness of the milk and scrupulous nature of the dairy workers. If Mary could not find certified raw milk, she was to boil it first. When traveling, Mary could mix powdered milk with boiled water. At one year the babies were to be weaned.

That was "scientific mothering." Today this term is widely derided. It has come to mean "overly precise, controlled." It has come to mean that doctors are in charge, not mothers. And it has come to mean ignorance. But baby care *should* be scientific, in my view. By that I mean that it should be evidence-based. And now the evidence tells us what Aunt Belle got wrong. Today we know that many mothers can nurse twins. We know there is no physiological reason to nurse babies on a fixed schedule. But the most glaring problem is that the formula served at Belle's hospital lacks essential fats, vitamins, and minerals. The recipe is a guess, and not a very good one. Making synthetic breast milk is harder than it looks.

In the 1950s, skeptics saw problems with formula, including its excessive burden on the kidneys and lack of essential fatty acids. Infant scurvy was still a problem, too, even though it was widely known since the 1920s, and by experts before that, that the vitamin C in raw milk or fresh juice would prevent it. As the pioneers of nutritionism had envisioned, experts met each problem in formula with a nutritional solution. Today formula contains vitamin C, omega-6 fats, and minerals, among many mandatory ingredients.

In 1959, iron-fortified formula appeared. Then as now, it was promoted vigorously to prevent anemia. But some experts, such as the pediatrician Michel Cohen, believe the benefits of supplemental iron are overstated. Iron-fortified formula may contain twenty times more iron than breast milk. The large dose is deliberate, because supplemental iron is poorly absorbed. Babies absorb only 4 percent of the iron in formula. As the concentration of iron in formula rises, absorption actually declines.[34]

Nor is it proven that extra iron helps babies. A study of more than eight hundred Chilean babies found that infants who were fed iron-fortified formula from six to twelve months had "significantly" lower developmental scores and "suggestively" lower IQ scores at age ten than infants getting less iron.[35] We know that iron interferes with zinc, which is vital for mental development. You will recall that inorganic iron feeds the wrong gut bacteria, which hobbles absorption of other nutrients.

Perhaps the most compelling argument against iron-fortified formula is that iron does not belong in the newborn diet. Your milk, and the milk of all mammals, lacks iron. In addition to being iron-poor, milk also contains lactoferrin, which ties up any random iron floating about. At first glance, this seems like an error, given that all living things need iron. With such a firm hand limiting the availability of iron to the nursling, we must suspect a deliberate strategy on nature's part.

Sure enough, there is logic in the missing iron. *E. coli*, the most common source of infant diarrhea in all species, depends on iron, as do other pathogens. As mentioned in the discussion of prenatal iron supplements, sequestering iron—keeping it out of the way of hungry microbes—is the body's response to infection. A low-iron diet protects newborns from iron-loving microbes. As iron expert Sharon Moalem described it to me, lactoferrin is like an armored truck: it transports iron safely to its destination, protecting it from marauding bacteria. Breast milk, in other words, is iron-poor by design. What iron it contains is easily absorbed by your baby.

Today many formulas contain synthetic fats attempting to mimic the ability of DHA and ARA in breast milk to feed the eye and brain. DHA and ARA can be derived from fish and egg yolks. In Europe, formula makers use fish. Here, Martek Biosciences makes a DHA substitute called DHASCO from the algae *Crypthecodinium cohnii*. Infant formula contains LA by law, so in theory, the infant can make ARA from it, but preterm babies can't do it well.[36] So Martek makes a synthetic ARA called ARASCO from the fungus *Mortierella alpina*. DHASCO and ARASCO are found in infant formula and many other food products, from soybean juice to "nutrition bars" and vegetarian supplements.

Do these imitation fats work for babies? The evidence is "mixed," reports the FDA. "Some studies in infants suggest that including these fatty acids in infant formulas may have positive effects on visual function and neural development over the short term," says a FDA fact sheet. "Other studies in infants do not confirm these benefits." So far, it appears that preterm babies may benefit, while the evidence for term babies is equivocal.[37] Formula with these oils causes digestive problems in some newborns.[38] We await long-term clinical trials.

"Milk remains a food of humbling complexity, to judge by the long, sorry saga of efforts to simulate it," Michael Pollan writes in his book *In Defense of Food*. "The entire history of baby formula has been the history of one overlooked nutrient after another: Liebig missed the vitamins and amino acids, and his successors missed the omega-3s . . . Even more than margarine, infant formula stands as the ultimate test product of nutritionism and a fair index of its hubris."

Don't misunderstand me. The government-regulated, scientifically derived, "nutritionally complete" infant formula you can buy is the closest we've come to a substance capable of doing a fraction of the considerable work of human milk. It keeps more babies alive than earlier versions of synthetic breast milk, recipes made in ignorance. We are wiser now. But our ignorance about the components of whole foods, and their dynamic effects in the human body, is not so easily banished. As good as formula is, it's not good enough.

The U.S. government estimates that in 1992, more than 8,100 newborns died because they did not receive breast milk.[39] If every baby were breast-fed for only twelve weeks, infant mortality in the United States—about 89,000 babies per year, one of the highest rates among rich countries—would decline by 5 percent.[40] According to the journal *Pediatrics*, 20 percent of deaths of babies one month to one year old could be prevented if every American baby got some breast milk.[41] Feeding formula exclusively in the first three months increases infant mortality by 60 percent.

The good news is that breast-feeding rates in the United States have climbed steadily since the nadir of the 1950s, when 20 percent of infants were breastfed. After a dip in the 1980s, the portion of babies getting any breast milk at birth rose to an historic high of 79 percent in 2011, according to the Centers for Disease Control, which asks mothers about baby feeding in (aptly) the National Immunization Survey. The 2012 and 2013 surveys found that at six months, 49 percent of babies born in 2011 were still nursing and 14 percent of babies were still getting breast milk at one year. The American Academy of Pediatrics recommends that breast-feeding continue for at least twelve months, and thereafter for as long as mother and baby desire. The World Health Organization recommends breast-feeding (alongside real food) for two years or longer.

## HEALTHY PEOPLE NURSING GOALS FOR 2020

| | |
|---|---|
| **Any Milk** | **82% of babies** |
| **Milk for 6 months** | **60% of babies** |
| **Milk for 1 year** | **34% of babies** |
| **Only breast milk only for 3 months** | **46% of babies** |
| **Only breast milk for 6 months** | **25% of babies** |
| **AAP advice** | **100% of babies for 12 months** |
| **WHO advice** | **100% of babies up to age two** |

SOURCE: *Centers for Disease Control and Prevention*

### WHEN YOU CANNOT NURSE YOUR BABY

I was lucky to nurse my baby, and easily at that. Other mothers nurse through pain, bleeding nipples, plugged ducts, abscesses, even biopsies. They nurse twins and triplets. Mothers nurse premature triplets in the intensive care unit by pumping milk which babies drink by tube. They nurse babies with cleft palates. Mothers with epilepsy and mothers who use wheelchairs nurse. Women who have one breast nurse. Mothers who have never been pregnant induce their milk supply to nurse the babies they adopt.

I was again lucky never to use a pump. For about a year, Julian was near me, and when I did leave him with the nanny to write this book, he was well on his way with other food and drink. I never even pumped milk for our twins. Many working mothers go back to work when the baby is six weeks old. Yet they still give their babies nothing but breast milk by pumping and freezing. They pump in cars and public bathrooms, in cockpits and boardrooms, plus less convenient, less private, and less hygienic places. They send breast milk with daddies, grandmothers, nannies, and day-care staff. They board planes and hail taxis toting breast milk. They keep it in insulated backbacks and hotel minibars.

These mothers amaze and humble me. I salute them. I also salute the CDC, which now includes ways to support nursing mothers in its 2014 Breast-feeding Report Card. Official practical support is long overdue.

A few mothers, no matter how dedicated, can't nurse at all. A woman may know in advance she cannot nurse for medical reasons. Or perhaps she encounters many obstacles, gets help, tries everything, and finally concludes that the baby needs more than she can give him. For these mothers, not being able to nurse, when so many able mothers feed formula instead, can be heartbreaking. I can only imagine it. If I had another baby and couldn't nurse for some reason, I'd be devastated. It's impossible to say what I would do.

Would I hire a wet nurse privately or ask a nursing mother to provide fresh milk? I noticed that a national employment agency, Certified Household Staffing, offers wet nurses. Only the Breast is an online matching service featuring wet nurses and frozen human milk. Maybe this traditional role is coming back. It certainly has a long history. Soranus, the pioneer in gynecology and pediatrics, explained how to choose a wet nurse in the first century.

Private arrangements between nursing women and mothers who cannot nurse are more common than you might think.[42] In the early nursing weeks, I often thought of my cesarean. I was haunted by mothers who come home from the hospital with milk but no baby to drink it, and by babies who come home with no mother. It still happens. With plenty of milk on my shirt and time on my hands, I considered finding a local baby who needed milk and offering to share, but never did anything about it.

More than a year later, I learned about Deidre Currie, a New Zealander and champion of real food. After a quick and sure romance over real food, she married American Archie Welch, settled in Michigan, started earning her nutrition degree, and with characteristic zeal planned a real food conference. Within months of the honeymoon, Deidre, thirty-eight, was pregnant and eating better than ever. The happy couple was planning a home birth, but instead Deidre ended up in the emergency room with a pulmonary embolism and the baby in distress. Though failing fast, she willed herself to hold on long enough to give birth to Jack, who weighed more than six pounds despite being six weeks early. Archie told me what happened.

> The word went out to mothers and they started pumping for him. His first meal in the hospital was breast milk from a mother who drove an hour and a half. She dropped off the milk, gave us all hugs, and left. She wouldn't accept any money for gas or anything. She said she was honored to help. All the mothers have been screened for diet, supplements, and drugs. About nine mothers consistently donate. I'm sure he's getting the advantage of a lot of different antibodies. As his appetite increases and some mums drop out, I've been adding raw cow milk. For a preemie, he is big. At four months, he is seventeen pounds and over two feet long. And happy. Jack is not a fussy child. Very calm, smiles a lot—but lets me know when he's hungry.

Deidre never saw or held her son. But she left him a legacy to last his entire life. In Jack's short life, many mothers have already cared for him. By way of thanks, Archie shares food with the nursing mothers. "I figure if the mothers are getting good fats and nutrients from healthy raw cow's milk, they will pass on those good things to Jack and to their own child. I also give them cod liver oil, coconut oil, meat, books, and my undying gratitude," he said. "What I do for them pales in comparison for what they do for Jack."

Jack was six months old when I met him. By then he was getting donated breast milk, raw cow milk, and a little egg yolk. He was a charming baby, in radiant health, strapping for his age. With his father's permission, I offered Jack my breast, and when he took it, Julian—then a toddler—got a funny look on his face. He was wide-eyed—and mad. He objected loudly and tried to swat the smaller baby away.

When mothers nurse each other's babies, it's called cross nursing. It can be handy when mothers are taking turns babysitting breast-fed babies or when a mother needs to take medicine. It can also help an adoptive mother who needs to increase her milk supply. An experienced nursing baby can latch on and get the milk supply going, leaving a breast ready for the adopted newborn. Cross nursing is neither common nor widely accepted. Attitudes range from complete acceptance to tepid tolerance to outrage. Even La Leche League doesn't recommend it.

Still, women do it. In a book of stories called *The Breastfeeding Café*, I read about Judy Wagner, a mother in Ithaca, New York, who was at wit's end, unable to nurse her daughter because of ruptured blood vessels, engorgement, a poor suckle, and other troubles. She turned to the nursing mothers she knew best. Two sisters drove hours to breast-feed their niece. The baby thrived, and by three months, mother and baby were a happy nursing pair. Grandmothers have nursed babies, even though they had no milk to offer.

Another choice is a human milk bank, where the milk is tested, pasteurized, frozen, and shipped to babies who need it. This used to be more common. In New York City, the Mother's Milk Bureau was open from 1921 to 1950. In 1937, it distributed more than five thousand quarts of pasteurized, frozen milk to six hundred babies. The bank paid nursing mothers thirteen cents an ounce plus a bus or streetcar ticket. Individuals bought it for thirty cents an ounce, hospitals paid twenty-five, and poor women got it free. The federal law that supported milk banks expired after World War II. Formula rapidly took over.

Milk banks are coming back. Today, babies who benefit from donor milk include premature infants in intensive care, babies failing on formula, twins and triplets, and adopted infants. Babies and toddlers with life-threatening diseases or conditions and children with failing immune systems or catastrophic diseases can get real milk. Mothers whose milk isn't suitable for consumption, because of disease or medications, also use milk banks.

Another option is homemade formula, according to a well-designed recipe. This is most demanding, because getting the formula right is an enormous responsibility. Yet babies are thriving on formula recipes devised with care by the Weston A. Price Foundation. The basic formula contains whole milk, whey, lactose, *Bifidobacterium infantis*, cream, cod liver oil, unrefined sunflower oil, extra-virgin olive oil, coconut oil, nutritional yeast, gelatin (for digestion), and acerola powder (for vitamin C). Unlike the formula you can buy, it's all real food. For babies who cannot drink cow milk, there are recipes with goat milk and meat.

If commercial formula is the only option, the best choice is an organic, low-iron cow milk formula in powder. (Liquid formula may contain a toxin called bisphenol A or BPA, which leaches from the container.) Soy formula is the worst choice. In 2008, the American Academy of Pediatrics reviewed the evidence on soy formula. The clear conclusion: Cow milk formula is superior.[43] "Soy protein is completely different from animal protein," says Dr. Frank Greer, chairman of the nutrition committee of the AAP. "Human infants are made to grow on animal protein." The AAP found that soy formula has no proven value in reducing colic or fussiness. If the baby is allergic to milk, the AAP recommends hypoallergenic cow milk formula. The only medical indication for soy formula is the rare metabolic disorder called galactosemia.

We've already discussed the all-important fats for brain development. Instead of buying formula with synthetic omega-6

## WHY I DON'T DRINK FORMULA

**The main ingredients in a milk-based formula are nonfat milk, soybean, coconut, and sunflower oil, lactose, rice starch, and maltodextrin. In a lactose-free formula, you'll find maltodextrin, sucrose, milk protein isolate, and safflower and soybean oil. A formula for babies who can't eat casein contains corn syrup as the main ingredient, plus soybean, coconut, and safflower oil, casein hydrosylate, and modified corn starch. The main ingredient in a soy formula is again corn syrup, followed by soy protein isolate, safflower oil, sugar, and soybean oil. The first ingredient in an organic soy formula is brown rice syrup. If you don't buy these ingredients, why should your baby eat them? The only real food here is coconut oil, which provides lauric acid, the antiviral fat found in breast milk.**

and omega-3 fats, give your baby real food. Your baby can eat gently cooked pastured egg yolks and a few drops of cod liver oil for ARA and DHA. A baby on formula would also benefit from eating a few other well-chosen, nutritious, and digestible foods, such as coconut oil and powdered beef or chicken broth, earlier than a breast-fed baby—say, at four or five months, instead of six or seven.

### CACHE OR CARRY?

Many new mothers are all aflutter about the actual business of breast-feeding. How often should I nurse? What if I don't make enough milk? Is my baby getting enough foremilk and hindmilk? Will breast-feeding hurt? Because most experts agree that breast is best, there is a stupendous quantity of information about breast-feeding in all sorts of places: books, Web sites, videos, pamphlets. Most of it is impressively thorough and professional. It's science-based. It's well written. And it's much, much more than you need to know.

When I was pregnant, I decided against the childbirth preparation classes. It seemed to me that my chief goal was to be physically fit, nutritionally stocked, and emotionally calm. The rest would take care of itself. But one class did interest me, and that was on breast-feeding. For although breast-feeding is natural, it is not always actually immediately obvious to the new mother how it's done. Nor is it necessarily automatic. Nursing is like a dance. It takes training and practice. It calls on both nature and nurture.

This is evident when you see confident nursing pairs only two weeks after birth. While you fumble around, as if you had six babies with eight mouths squirming in your lap, these mothers are nursing effortlessly, all while balancing coffee cups, talking on the phone, switching sides, and smiling. Once mastered, nursing is not easily forgotten. You know this when you see the mother of a toddler in late pregnancy, blithely carrying on with mothering, cooking, work, and play. The last thing she needs is a lesson.

But you might. Some specific maneuvers make breast-feeding much easier. Without them, you flail around a bit. Without them, you may even fail—at least at first. The baby doesn't get a good latch, she's hungry, and you feel like a flop. These bits are most easily explained, and grasped by the first-timer, when a woman who has nursed a few babies, and watched a few hundred other babies nurse, shows you how to go about it, either by letting you hold her baby or with a life-size baby doll. Ask mothers you know. Failing that, hire a professional.

So, one evening I found myself in a breast-feeding class and getting very cross. The atmosphere was serious, as if we were getting instructions for an emergency water landing. Whether the instructor set the tone, or the nervous parents, I couldn't say. Rather like most prenatal advice, the information fell in two categories: a long list of things to remember and an equally long list of thing that can go wrong. I gritted my teeth, deciding more than once not to leave early. Three hours later, I was glad I waited for my turn with the doll, which was surprisingly useful, but gladder to leave, and gladder still I'd skipped the other childbirth classes.

Much later, long after I'd figured out how to breast-feed my own baby, I realized what I was looking for that evening: the proverbial big picture. What is the key to successful breast-feeding? Not the tips and techniques—the big idea. Even though I'd been taught the maneuvers in class, in the hospital by a lactation consultant, at La Leche League meetings, and by my mother, the early days still found me wailing loudly, "Why is breast-feeding so *difficult*?"

I wish I'd known then what I've figured out since. Nursing your baby is not about understanding hindmilk or breast capacity, the cross-cradle hold or the letdown reflex. We *Homo sapiens* think too much. Blame the fish oil in our oversized neocortex.

The key to successful breast-feeding is to act like the mammal you are. If you can do that, things will probably go smoothly. I'm also confident you will worry less. Even the authors of breast-feeding manuals, amid the biological science and technical tips, remind us that too much information can backfire.

So, one warning: We won't deal here with breast-feeding problems—not even common ones, like sore nipples. My reasons are philosophical and practical. Above all, I want to encourage you, and reading about things that can go wrong will merely fill your head with problems you're unlikely to have. Furthermore, if you do have trouble, specific advice from someone who watches you nurse will be much more helpful than my general advice from a thousand miles away. Go to a La Leche League meeting or call a postpartum doula or lactation consultant to your house. It will be time or money well spent. What's not wise is to struggle alone, feeling like a lousy mother because you "cannot" feed your baby. Of course you can. A monkey can do it.

So can the hyena, possum, and lemur—but they all go about it differently. Mammals and their mammary glands come in all shapes and sizes. Unlike the small, droopy sacks monkeys sport, our mammary glands are permanently swollen, more so when we nurse. A whale mammary gland is five feet long and weighs 250 pounds. The porcupine has no nipple. Milk oozes from ducts into indentations in her skin, where babies lap it up. The Tammar Wallaby crawls into his mother's pouch, partially swallows his personal teat, and hangs on to it for several months. The teat and gland respond to his suckle and develop as he grows. There are many ways to deliver milk to babies.

Now we come to the interesting—and helpful—part. Mammals also care for their babies in different ways. The South African animal biologist Nils Bergman described four mothering styles, according to the kind of milk the mother makes. Mothers whose milk is thin never leave their babies. They carry them everywhere and nurse often. Bergman called them "carry" mothers. Mothers with rich milk stash the babies in a safe place and then leave, often for many hours. These he called "cache" mothers. The two other styles are somewhere in between.

Without a doubt, you are a "carry" mother. Your baby cannot walk. She cannot even roll over. She very much needs to be carried. She is also fairly skinny, with no fur and no means of clothing herself. She cannot even coordinate her arms to pull a blanket over her little body. She relies on the warmth of your body. It's no accident that your milk has the lowest levels of fat and protein of any mammal. Your baby needs to stay near you so she can drink your thin milk when she's hungry, which is often.

To me, this analysis of mothering habits and milk recipes was vivid. It helped me see what I had to do. It helped me turn down my neocortex—it's difficult to turn off—and stop thinking about nursing technique. It helped me put ignorant comments where they belonged. ("Won't you spoil him by holding him and nursing all the time?") It helped me surrender my old life, at

## WHAT KIND OF MAMMAL ARE YOU?

- *Cache* mammals, such as the deer or rabbit, hide their young, which are mature at birth, and return to see them infrequently, about every twelve hours. Their milk is high in protein and fat to keep the babies going in the long time between meals.

- *Nest* mammals include the dog and cat. Less mature at birth, kittens and puppies stay cozy in a nest, and their mother visits several times daily. Her milk contains less protein and fat than cache mammal milk.

- *Follow* mammals, such as the giraffe and cow, have mature babies that can walk behind their mothers. Because babies are able to feed frequently, their milk contains still less fat and protein than cache or nest milk.

- *Carry* mammals include the kangaroo and primates. Babies are helpless at birth. They must be carried constantly. They cannot regulate body temperature. They feed round the clock on milk with relatively little fat and protein. That's your baby.

least temporarily, in order to be the mother nature intended. It helped me ask for help. (It's harder for carry mammals to shop for food, cook supper, and wash the dishes.)

If birth is still ahead of you, try to set the stage for nursing. The best beginning is a physiologically normal birth. When the mother gets narcotics, babies don't nurse as easily. When babies are born by cesarean, nursing is delayed. As I know well, you cannot control how your baby is born. Still, it's worth aiming for the optimal outcome. Lots of skin-to-skin contact, warmth, darkness, and privacy will help you nurse earlier and more easily, even after a cesarean. Early nursing has several benefits for mother and baby. It will make you more confident, sooner. It will stimulate prolactin receptors, which establishes a good milk supply. In the baby, early breast-feeding clears meconium faster, reduces temporary jaundice, and regulates blood sugar.

Things will be much easier if you nurse on cue, which merely means that you nurse when the baby asks. That will be often. You may feel like a slave to nursing in the early days. You are. But it makes things much smoother, and it's temporary. Later—probably in just a few weeks—life will be more flexible. There will be longer intervals between feedings, and you will be the expert of your baby's rhythms. Right now, your newborn needs you nearby and responsive. She sets the schedule. Don't even try to guess what it is. Just follow along. In the 1950s, bottle-feeding was thought to be superior because it was precise and quantifiable. Breast-feeding is neither. And still it's better than any other way to feed babies.

The most basic reason to nurse on cue is physiological. In the very beginning, you're making one to three ounces of colostrum per day—a trickle. Small and frequent sips maximize the colostrum your baby gets. Also, her tiny stomach fills up fast and empties just as quickly. One little poop later, and she's ravenous. Milk satisfies her thirst. She won't drink water for six months. You wouldn't want to drink water on a schedule, so why should your baby?

Psychological reasons to nurse on cue are also compelling. As you will soon know, your baby wants to be near you. This desire is called "attachment." Attachment behavior—crying, clinging, whimpering, wriggling, smiling, and (eventually) following—has one purpose in the infant—to maintain physical proximity to his mother, or to any main caregiver, including fathers, adoptive parents, and nannies. In the 1950s, the British psychologist John Bowlby explained that the survival instincts of the infant demand that he act this way. The infant who does not insist on staying close is less likely to thrive. His physical health depends on it.

So does his emotional health. In the 1950s and 1960s, the American psychologist Harry Harlow did experiments with baby

monkeys showing the importance of attachment for its own
sake. He separated baby monkeys from their mothers and gave
them mother substitutes made of wire. One wire doll was
"friendly." Covered with soft terry cloth, she was nice to cling
to, but offered no food. The other mother was plain wire, but
she did bear a nipple with milk. The monkeys spent most of
their time hugging the soft mother and only darted over to the
wire mother to feed. Just like monkeys, human babies feel a
strong need to be near their mothers, food or no food, and they
prefer nice, cozy mothers to cold, hostile ones.

When infants lose contact with their mothers—or their
mothers are erratic or unresponsive—babies suffer psychologi-
cally. They are less secure, less independent, and (paradoxically)
more clingy. They're also sad. Depression is a complex condition
with multiple causes—genetic, nutritional, seasonal, conditional—
but it's simple to create experimental depression in animals:
separate the newborn from its mother. Depression is miserable
indeed. It can also make you sick. In the depressed creature,
noradrenaline and serotonin drop and stress hormones rise. "In
a baby or young child a raised level of cortisol has a spectacular
effect in reducing the size of the thymus," writes Odent in *Primal Health*. As you'll recall, this gland is central to immunity.

The baby tries to get close, and the mother responds. This
describes mother-baby habits for most of human history. Researchers compared mothering in 176 nonindustrial societies to
mothering in American culture. "Whether measured by body
contact, sleeping distance, response to crying, or weaning age,
mother-infant contact and maternal indulgence of infants appeared to be less in the United States than in the broad
cross-cultural range," they found. According to the Stone Age
expert S. Boyd Eaton, mothers have been keeping babies close
for tens of millions of years.

You don't have to live in a traditional culture to act like a
traditional mother. You just hold your baby a lot, respond when
she cries, carry your baby in a sling or other carrier, and sleep

together—if not in the same bed, in the same room. I'm glad these time-honored habits are coming back with American mothers and fathers. "The environment of the newborn is the parent: not the crib, bassinet, playpen, car seat, stroller, bouncy seat," writes Erica Lyon in *The Big Book of Birth*. "Our compulsions to check on the baby and have the baby close to us are *normal*." You're not neurotic, and you're not indulgent. You're a carry mammal.

Consider the baby's perspective. All he knows is that the world is dangerous and that you are his lifeline. "A screaming baby alone in its cot or lined up with rows of other screaming newborns is a neglected baby," says Sheila Kitzinger, the English baby expert. "He cannot know that help is near, that milk is coming in half an hour, or twenty minutes, or even five minutes. He cannot know that loving arms are waiting to hold him. He is to all intents and purposes completely isolated and abandoned." This doesn't mean you can never get a break to eat or take a shower. All your baby needs to know is that *someone* who cares is nearby and will respond.

Your reward for all this hard work now is a confident and healthy toddler and child. Separation and independence will come in time. When is that? It's coming already, right under your nose. Babies are very different at three months, and six, and nine. Sometime between one and three, your baby starts to be more confident on her own and to form tighter attachments to persons other than you. Right now, that may seem to be a long time away. Mothers told me it would whiz by. Now I know it's true.

There is also an immediate benefit. Life with a newborn will be much easier if you make yourself available to your baby most of the time. Never mind being a "good" mother; I found it much easier for *me* to surrender to Julian rather than to resist or wish away his calls. Everything about baby care, including nursing, is less taxing when you stay close and respond quickly.

Night-nursing, which all newborns need, is much easier when you sleep with your baby. He can sleep in your bed or in a little caboose, called a co-sleeper, next to yours. When he cries, you don't have to rouse yourself to walk down the hall to the nursery. Instead, a delicate little dance takes place for night-feeds. The baby makes small noises and works his way over to you. You move a bit to accommodate him. Now he's nursing. Mother, baby, and father—if he woke up at all—are soon back to sleep.

Today there is a wealth of information about co-sleeping. With a little research, you can easily satisfy yourself that it's safe, except in certain conditions, such as when the mother or father is too drunk to be aware of the sleeping infant. With young babies, I'm a fan of the family bed, and so were Julian and Rose, but it's not for every parent, and our son Jacob preferred to sleep and nap on his own from the beginning. Of all the good reasons to sleep with your wakeful or hungry baby, my favorite was getting more sleep. I was a sleepy mammal.

## TIPS AND MYTHS

Many first-time mothers have the most basic fears about nursing. Here's one: What if I can't tell when my baby is hungry? Don't worry. You'll figure out the cues for "feed me" in short order. For a newborn there are few other requests. They mostly come down to *sleepy* (help me sleep), *uncomfortable* (change my diaper), and *hungry* (nurse me). Now that we understand attachment, we can add *lonely* (hold me).

Newborns tell you all this with noises and gestures. Typical nursing cues are rooting—turning her head from side to side, mouth wide open—putting her hand to her mouth, and fussing. There are also fairly specific sounds, if not words exactly. According to some newborn "language" experts, the hungry one is sort of a "nyeh" sound.[44] By the time I learned that, Julian was clearly requesting "baba." Still, even without formal training, I figured out when Julian was hungry. "He has a couple of cries," I noted after about a month. "Sucking knuckles, wrist, forearm; tongue in and out; mewling; hands to face; hands reaching out to me, if in arms=wants to nurse. If he's [very] hungry, it will escalate to full crying, and doesn't stop if I don't come." These were distinguishable from the loud and sudden "pee" cry—has to pee or just did—and from the "pay attention" or "hurry up" cry.

Watch the baby, not the clock. There is no schedule for a breast-fed baby. She knows when she is hungry. You need only sit down and nurse. Patterns may emerge, of course. As a newborn, Julian nursed nearly every night at one A.M., no matter when we went to sleep. Like many babies, he also wanted to nurse a lot, off and on, between six and nine P.M. This is called "cluster feeding." There's nothing to know about it except that it's not a good time to cook dinner, check e-mail, or wash your hair. We spent some tearful evenings burning supper before I realized this. The cluster hour is a great time to sit in the nursing chair with a book or the phone. If someone can bring you a bowl of food and fill your water glass, that's nice.

There is a wide range of healthy nursing patterns. Most babies nurse eight to twelve times in twenty-four hours. The more often, the better. You will produce more milk, the baby will gain weight, and your breasts will not be uncomfortably full. Try to nurse at an early cue, before the baby is desperate. A hysterically hungry baby has more trouble latching on and relaxing. When we went walking and stayed out too long, Julian would be strung out when we finally sat down to nurse, at, say, four or five P.M., and then he would drink too fast and throw up. It was not unreasonable to blame myself for these episodes.

Nursing is your full-time job. Not for all time. Just now. In the early days you may well spend eight hours—half your waking day—in the nursing chair, either preparing to nurse, trying to nurse, nursing, or wrapping up. That's normal. Just get ready to abandon your old routine. Trying to keep to a rigid schedule is sure to end in tears—yours.

Now we turn to the promised technical advice. You and your baby must figure out the "latch." Don't worry. It's not a piece of artisanal carpentry. It's just a little arrangement for two people. It's not so different from learning to spoon with someone you love. At first you're awkward, but pretty soon you're doing it in your sleep. In a short time, you will be getting latches like old hands. But at the beginning, the latch can be challenging.

What does it mean? Simply this: The baby is properly attached to your breast. Notice I said "breast," not "nipple." One key to successful latches—that means comfortable and milk producing—is that the baby's upper and lower palate grab your whole breast or quite a lot of it. The baby's lips should not be nipping at your nipple. Sucking on the nipple alone will hurt you and produce very little milk, frustrating everyone.

Even if you struggle with latches at first, carry on. They will come. This was the most discouraging part for me. Perhaps it had to do with the drugs we got. After a natural birth, some mothers and babies lock eyes within minutes. Julian didn't look at me directly until seven hours after he was born. A baby born without drugs may climb up her mother's belly, root for the nipple, and latch on in minutes or hours, but suckling is delayed by hours after surgery.[45]

After a cesarean, levels of prolactin and oxytocin are lower. Oxytocin causes the little muscles in the alveoli to contract, pushing milk through the ducts and out the pinholes in the nipple. During the "letdown," you may feel warmth, tingling, or a gentle ache. The immediate effects of reduced prolactin and delayed nursing are usually not serious. The baby gets less milk and gains weight less quickly. Note that some weight loss after birth is normal. Still, twice as many babies born naturally (40 percent) regain their birth weight in six days as cesarean babies (20 percent). In some cases, the baby may never get breast milk. Breast-feeding rates are significantly lower after a cesarean.

Julian nibbled and sucked at my nipple, the colostrum dribbling out as it's meant to, but he didn't get a latch or any milk until nearly two days after he was born. Not that we didn't try.

We practiced a lot. After the first thrilling latch, we tried some more. We sometimes tried for thirty minutes to get a latch. I felt like crying and did. There were many frustrating night-feedings, while a foggy Nina and a hungry Julian tried and tried to nurse. I had to turn the light on, get out the props, sit up, and give it my full attention. On the eleventh day, we began to get latches easily. Sooner or later, you will, too.

I was following what was then the standard technical advice about how to breast-feed. I sat up, holding Julian in a perpendicular fashion across my waist. He faced me in a position known as "nose to nipple, tummy to tummy." Ideally, he rested across a firm pillow, so that I did not need to hold him up in the air. (The pillow functions like those platforms window washers attach to skyscrapers: you are the skyscraper, and you are slippery. Holding the baby against gravity, with her legs dangling mid-air, your arms and shoulders quickly tire. A pillow also keeps you upright, which is helpful when things go badly; the more you fail, the more you hunch, lean, lurch, and grip the poor baby.) Thus arranged, I tickled his lower lip with my nipple, which triggers the mouth to open wide, like that of a hungry baby bird, and pressed quickly and firmly on his back, hoping that his mouth would land directly around the nipple and form a suction, otherwise known as the latch.

You will know immediately when you've got it. You'll feel a gentle suction. It might feel funny at first. The breast is deep in your baby's mouth, which is doing some highly precise mechanical movements involving her hard and soft palate and tongue, movements which maximize milk flow and stimulate milk production. (The mechanics have been described by smart people in complex equations.) The muscles in her cheek and jaw are working. You may spot a little throbbing in her temple. You will see and hear her swallowing. *Glug, glug.* Hurrah!

One more thing. She will stay there. A bad latch is a short-lived latch. The baby will come off, root again, keep trying. You will repeat the steps above, probably many times. Julian and I certainly did. With Rose and Jacob, I took the same approach. And things were much easier, for several reasons now clear in hindsight. One, Julian was a cesarean baby, which can cause early difficulty with latches. Two, I had more experience. Three, Julian (as we discovered around his third birthday) has several gross and fine motor delays, which made coordinating the various physical maneuvers required much more challenging for him. Nevertheless, after days of struggle, we had a trouble-free nursing career lasting two years.

That said, if I were to have another baby, I'd try something else, something new in the trade with the friendly moniker "laid-back breast-feeding." The mother reclines and the baby lies on her chest, in line with her body; that's the laid-back part. This approach, which midwife and lecturer Suzanne Colson is slowly making famous, has two chief advantages. First, it makes the most of gravity. Lying on the mother's chest, the baby stays near his mother without either party's effort. Second, this position appears to release up to twenty primitive neonatal reflexes (PNRs), powerful forces that serve the nursing pair by promoting easy latches.

Healthy babies are born with a few dozen PNRs. A famous one is the "startle reflex." When surprised, the baby throws her arms out wide, as if to hug someone or something. Other reflexes involve putting the hand to the mouth, leg-cycling, grasping, and rolling. Two PNRs related to breast-feeding are the rooting (mouth twitches, head moves side to side) and sucking reflexes. Colson and her colleagues studied PNRs in nursing pairs in both positions: tummy-to-tummy or laid-back. "Results clearly demonstrated a statistically significant difference: more reflexes were released as stimulants when the mothers lay back than when they sat upright or lay on their sides," she wrote in the 2012 issue of *Midwifery Today*. When researchers observed the perpendicular position I used, PNRs sometimes thwarted latches. "The more the mother struggled to elicit mouth gape, leading in with the chin, the tighter she gripped the baby's back.

The firmer the grip, the more the baby struggled with frantic arm and/or leg cycling PNRs, increasing in strength and amplitude as he worked himself up to a crying state." In the laid-back position, by contrast, "babies often latched on without help."

Colson named her method "biological nurturing," implying that breast-feeding is part nature and part nurture. "Midwives have always believed that the maternal body is specifically designed for pregnancy and spontaneous birth," she wrote. "The double entendre in laid-back breastfeeding suggests that we can be relaxed and confident after the birth as well."

And then, one day, breast-feeding will be easy. You'll look like you've been at it for years. Like giraffes, whales, and wallabies, you and your baby are wired to nurse. But you won't know how until you try. To keep your head clear, here are a few things *not* to worry about.

*The baby's mouth must cover your areola.* Maybe it will, maybe it won't. Whether the dark part of your nipple is visible with a good latch depends on the size of your breast, areola, and baby. A good mouthful of breast will be in there, but that looks very different from breast to breast.

*Make sure the baby gets enough skim and cream.* Foremilk, which comes out first, is the skim. Hindmilk, which follows, contains more fat and protein. Babies like skim when they're thirsty and cream when they're hungry. They need both to grow, but don't worry about it. If you empty each breast from time to time throughout the day, that's fine.

*You must empty both sides at each nursing.* Or was I supposed to empty *one* breast at each nursing? I never could follow this one. My right breast was bigger. I assumed this was a problem. I assumed he was not emptying it properly. Then I assumed he emptied it too often, so the milk supply was growing too fast on the right and shrinking on the left. I made sure he'd empty the left side first, then the right. I started him on the breast he'd nursed last. I only read about some of the other tips. I didn't try them, because they were hard to remember and the ones I tried didn't work. Rules make you think; I needed to be in mammal mode. As for my large breast, it never changed. Many women are lopsided.

*Don't forget to burp!* Burping your baby to release air in her belly was important when babies were fed with bottles. It's less important with nursing on cue, because a breast-fed baby doesn't overeat. A gentle tap on the back can help, especially when the latch isn't solid and the baby seems to be getting more air than milk. But you may not hear anything exciting.

*You don't have enough milk.* First you may worry that your milk isn't coming. It may take a few days, but it's coming. When it does, there will be no mistaking it. Your breasts will look and feel very different. A true inadequate milk supply is extremely rare. If your milk supply is low, the cure is always the same: hydration, good food, and more time nursing. The more you nurse, the more milk you make. For increasing your milk supply, pumping exclusively is not as good as letting the baby suckle. If you seem to have too much milk, just wait. It will adjust to your baby's appetite.

*Your breasts are too small or empty.* There is no such thing. Small and large breasts both produce plenty of milk to feed a baby. Your breasts are never empty. The minute your baby starts to suck, the mammary gland starts making milk. About 90 percent of breast milk is produced from your diet and your fat. The other 10 percent is manufactured right in the mammary gland.

*The baby is not getting enough milk.* There is no need to log mountains of data on how long your baby is on the breast. All you need to see are pees and poops. Babies are born a little waterlogged. That's one reason most babies lose weight in the first week. Over a slightly longer period, weight gain is the gold standard for whether the baby is eating well. The doctor or midwife can tell you if your baby is gaining enough.

*Your baby is too sleepy.* This was the discussion that nearly made me walk out of the nursing class. You could see exactly what the terrified parents were thinking. *My baby will starve to death in her sleep, and it will be my fault.* All newborns sleep a lot in the first few days. Every new baby, however he was born, has been through quite a journey. Babies can survive on nutrient stores and dribbles of colostrum until your milk comes in.

Very rarely, a baby is the sleepy type. It happens more often with newborn jaundice, when the liver, which doesn't work properly for several days, cannot completely flush bilirubin, a by-product of the breakdown of hemoglobin, from the blood. The buildup of bilirubin makes the skin slightly yellow. The treatment is sunlight and breast-feeding, which will empty the baby's bowels.

Sometimes, a sleepy baby gets sleepier. In such cases, a lactation consultant may suggest you wake him to nurse. Please file this under Not Likely. It would be odd indeed if babies were too sleepy to eat. Carry mammal babies wake up frequently to fill their tiny stomachs. Of course they do. Otherwise, new mothers and fathers wouldn't be bleary-eyed. What a funny world that would be.

# CHAPTER 5
# First Foods

## EAST OF EDEN

I was not in a hurry for Julian to start eating real food. It was not that I wanted to breast-feed forever. I didn't. It was not that I enjoyed Julian's total dependence on me and no one else. I didn't. When he started to last for longer stretches without nursing, I was delighted. Things were more flexible. But most of all, I didn't feel quite so much like a bucket of milk on two legs. I loved getting a babysitter, rummaging in the back of the closet for a dress I couldn't nurse in, and going out with Rob.

But there was something utopian about nursing. My breasts met Julian's nutritional needs. Anywhere we went, I carried his breakfast, lunch, dinner, and snacks in the perfect container. I didn't have to think. Julian was eight months old when we went on tour to promote the paperback edition of *Real Food*. Travel was a breeze. I didn't have to buy, pack, cook, or wash anything. Long flights, short ones, delays, bad hotel food, time zone changes—none of it mattered. There was nothing to take, spill, or spoil. Extreme conditions were no problem. On a windy sand dune or a desert hike in the blazing sun, Julian didn't even need water. I had it. Nursing was a kind of Eden.

I knew mothers who felt the opposite. Whether they liked nursing or not, they were looking forward to baby's first fistful of banana, first slurp of boiled carrot. They couldn't wait to make baby food and freeze little portions in ice cube trays. I've read baby food cookbooks in which mother and father enthuse about fortnightly purée-and-freeze parties. They are justly proud and say they're having a fine old time. I believe them.

That's not me. Quite apart from the extra work—shopping, cooking, and cleaning for another person on two legs, another set of taste buds—I saw beyond the hedgerows of our green Eden a whole mess of choices. I am happy to tackle what Paul Rozin called the Omnivore's Dilemma for myself. I know pretty much what's good for my species and for my own body. I can make my way around the supermarket, even with all those misleading labels. I know what to eat.

But making all the decisions for our ever-plumper son was daunting. I was leery of wandering East of Eden, nutritionally speaking. It seemed like a heavy responsibility for one imperfect woman, and I didn't want to screw up. What should Julian eat? The God of Infant Nutrition wasn't talking, so I fell back on a combination I respect, namely one part tradition, one part science, and a pinch of common sense. You'll have to dip into your own supply of good sense, but here's a bit of science and tradition to consider.

In the 1920s and 1930s, a pioneering midwestern pediatrician named Clara Davis and her team of nurses set out a range of foods for infants and let them eat anything they wanted, every day, for months.[1] The complete smorgasbord included broiled ground beef and lamb; steamed and minced haddock, chicken, sweetbreads, brains, liver, and kidneys; broiled beef and veal bone marrow; bone jelly (or reduced veal stock); raw and poached eggs; steel-cut oats, ground whole wheat, cornmeal, and whole barley (all boiled); raw oats and wheat; rye crackers; raw apples, bananas, oranges, pineapple, and peaches; steamed apples; baked bananas; raw tomatoes, lettuce, carrots, cabbage, and peas; steamed beets, carrots, peas, turnips, cauliflower, cabbage, and spinach; and baked potatoes. The babies could drink water, whole milk, cultured milk, and sometimes fresh orange juice. Each baby had his own small dish of sea salt.

The foods alone made Davis a renegade. Scientific mothering was in full flower. Doctors were in charge of child nutrition, and they had fixed ideas. "Children were allotted certain foods on a strict schedule and then only in small quantities," says the pediatrician Benjamin Scheindlin. In the 1920s, doctors recommended a precise sequence: sieved vegetable soup at one year, potato at eighteen months, and other vegetables at age two.[2] Bananas were considered indigestible.

Davis called this a "prescription of diet by limitation," and she was skeptical. Unable to find any research to justify it, she set about collecting her own data about baby food. She called it the "self-selection of diet experiment." Bucking the advice of her fellow doctors, Davis greatly expanded the menu and let the babies eat anything they wanted. She and her nurses gave no instructions, no encouragement, and no discouragement. The babies were to eat what they liked—no more, no less.

Her research protocol was meticulous. Each meal included grains, a couple of meats, and fruits and vegetables. Every dish was unseasoned and unmixed; that is, there were no recipes. Instead of meatloaf, babies got beef in one bowl and carrots in another, the better to measure consumption. Each baby ate alone, which ruled out imitation as a factor. He could use his fingers or a spoon, as he wished. A nurse sat with each baby during the meal but did not offer any food. If the baby wanted more, he had to ask or gesture, and the nurse would refill the dish without comment. Every food was weighed, including spilled food, and careful records of consumption were kept.

What happened? The babies had varied and good appetites. At a given meal, choices could be extreme. One baby ate mostly bone marrow; another regularly drank a quart of milk with lunch. One baby ate seven eggs in one day and another, four bananas, while one occasionally took handfuls of salt. Yet they didn't get stomachaches or otherwise suffer from these odd meals. Food jags lasting for days were common. A boy named Donald, always a fruit lover, had a brief lust for oranges, peaking at nearly two pounds daily. But over time, all the babies ate a varied diet, including much more meat than doctors recommended. As for the notorious pickiness of the typical toddler, "it did not rear its head in Dr. Davis's nursery," says Scheindlin.

Most revealing, all the children thrived. Analysis of more than thirty-six thousand meals showed that the babies, who were mostly breast-fed orphans, were well nourished. Their meals not only met but exceeded known nutritional needs. In fact, the babies seemed to know what they were doing. A nine-month-old boy with rickets drank cod liver oil until his rickets was cured, then ignored it. In short, the Clara Davis babies contradicted most of the advice doctors were giving mothers—if not all of it.

There is, of course, a blemish of reality in this utopian food story. Davis herself knew it, and you probably know it, too. Babies wouldn't find it so easy to eat a wholesome and balanced diet for months on end if the tray also had junk food on it. "She tells how primitive people, like children, choose well-balanced diets from native foods, but when highly processed foods are introduced, appetites fail to guide and digestive troubles and nutritional deficiencies ensue," wrote the psychologist Niles Newton in *The Family Book of Child Care*.

Don't we know it. Healthy eating is all in the foods you give your baby. We have to try to avoid the siren song of white flour and sugar in our own kitchen, on our block, in restaurants, on planes—in the real world.

Still, these famous experiments leave us something valuable: a list of good foods. Arrogant pediatricians, absorbed in their own unscientific recommendations, paid their innovative colleague a back-handed compliment. "Of course your children thrive," they said dismissively. "The foods you give them are foolproof."

When I was growing up, Clara Davis was a household hero. My mother took her baby-feeding advice wholly from Davis, via her disciple Adelle Davis. Mom was careful to provide nutritious foods and to avoid commentary at meals. It suited me as a child, and later, as a grown woman, it still made sense. All my life, I dreamed of doing for my own baby what the Clara Davis nurses did for those orphans. If nothing else, I could start with a list of foolproof foods. Now you have the list.

## READINESS IS ALL

I know the First Supper is momentous, but there is really very little to think about. Babies are ready for real food between five and nine months. Four months is early and ten months is late, but neither is unheard of in healthy breast-fed babies.

When is *your* baby ready? She is ready when she can sit up on her own. This indicates a certain control of her trunk. Her mouth and throat are stronger and more coordinated. When you put food on her tongue, she does not immediately eject it. This milestone has a technical description. It's said that "the tongue thrust has resolved." But you needn't be more than a casual observer on this point. When Julian ate his first foods, he stuck out his tongue plenty. Yet he was clearly relishing and swallowing food.

Your baby may have teeth, and she may not. Teeth have nothing to do with readiness to eat. You can verify this by sticking your finger where her molars will be. She can flatten all sorts of things back there, thanks to the bone under her gums. In any case, slicing (with sharp teeth) and chewing (with broad molars) are not the point. That comes later. New flavors and textures are the point.

Your baby may be big or small, trim or chubby. She may sleep through the night or wake up to nurse. She may reach for your food, but that's not important either. She's interested in anything you're busy with, whether it's your keys or your coffee. She probably puts anything she can grasp into her mouth already. You wouldn't try first foods when your breast-fed baby is vomiting or has diarrhea, but such things are common sense.

That's it. There are no other general considerations worth mentioning.

There is no need to rush the first meal. Nor is there any nutritional reason to delay it artificially if the baby is breast-fed. Julian tasted a few foods before he was six months old. Once Rob put fresh orange juice to his lips. At five months, he gnawed on a banana, but nothing went down. He had a sip of water. When I mentioned the water to a La Leche League leader, she told me that I couldn't describe Julian as exclusively breast-fed at six months. For a moment, I felt sad, as if I'd lost the Gold Medal for Exclusive Breast-feeding. The next moment, I thought, *What arrant nonsense!*

Modern advice about exclusive breast-feeding, good as it is, got me thinking. Extended nursing is certainly good for babies and drinking formula isn't. But it's not clear that delaying good food is as important. Traditionally, mothers probably nursed longer and gave real food earlier than we do. They gave babies easily digestible, nutritious foods, such as fish, liver, eggs, fruit, and sweet potatoes, sometimes prechewed.[3]

Official opinion varies about when to offer complementary foods, but not so much that it matters. The World Health Organization says four to six months, while the American Academy of Pediatricians says six. The fact is that few good studies have looked closely at this. I read them. What they all underscore is the importance of a decent diet. Babies weaned to nutrient-poor foods don't thrive. We know that. But when you start matters little. Don't get hung up on how old your baby is. If you nurse a long time and give your baby good food, he'll grow. While he's experimenting, nursing is the great equalizer. Breast milk gives your baby a steady stream of complete nutrition during the sloppy transition to real food.

## BABY FOODS

It seemed to me that you'd find the best advice about first foods from books written before ready-made baby food became widely available. Mothers had to keep their babies alive on tradition and good sense, without the benefit of "scientifically proven" and commercially driven recipes. So I checked with good old Aunt Belle. Circa 1921, she recommended milk, lamb and chicken broth, poached eggs, and beef "juice," made by grinding and squeezing a lightly broiled steak, all with a pinch of salt. Good advice. Note that these foods are whole, simple, and homemade.

Baby physiology suggests why meat, fish, and eggs are good first foods. The infant stomach has abundant digestive agents for protein and fats, including the enzyme pepsin and hydrochloric acid, plus a special enzyme for absorbing cholesterol. But babies don't make amylase, which breaks down starch, for about a year, so any carbohydrate must be easy to digest. As we'll see, cereals don't qualify.

Aunt Belle was not afraid of a little salt. Your baby's body contains about fourteen grams of this vital food. He uses it for metabolism, detoxification, shuttling nutrients around, and optimal hormone, immune, and nervous function. Chloride is necessary to form glial cells in the brain. But don't rely on standard table salt. It's pure sodium chloride. Whole salt has more than eighty essential minerals and trace elements, including iodine, potassium, magnesium, and sulfur.

Like the Clara Davis babies, your baby can eat unrefined sea salt to taste. Our children ate meat, fish, eggs, and vegetables with real salt from the start. If his food is already salty, such as Romano cheese or salmon roe, I don't add more. Now and then I let them put a finger in the salt or offered a coarse lump to suck on. As with any food, if they didn't want it, they didn't eat it. Choosing salt (or not) is just another part of learning about flavor, appetite, and thirst.

If you start early—before six months—I recommend lightly cooked egg yolk with a pinch of salt, a little cod liver oil, and banana. These brain foods are easy for the baby stomach to handle. We've talked about the vital fats and vitamins in eggs and cod liver oil. Tasty and soft, the banana contains its own amylase. It's an unusually fine plant source of vitamin $B_6$, which helps create neurotransmitters, including serotonin, melatonin, and dopamine. I'm a big fan of whole milk.

After six months, just about any real food is good. Babies can start with meat, poultry, fish, eggs, dairy, any fruits and vegetables, and traditional fats—namely butter, olive oil, and coconut oil. Whole milk, buttermilk, yogurt, cheese, cottage cheese, and sour cream are great foods. So are fresh coconut and coconut milk, which (like your milk) contain immune-boosting lauric acid. Avocado chunks with olive oil and salt make a wonderful baby dish, soft to gum and rich in vitamin E.

That should get things under way. I offer no recipes because I didn't use any. Keep it light and playful. Don't think too much. "Some child-rearing books would have you believe that introducing your baby to solid foods is a risky scientific experiment," says the ever-sensible Dr. Michel Cohen. "These books are full of frivolous warnings that could drive any parent crazy." When in doubt, refer to the real food rule—if we've been eating it for a few thousand years, it's probably OK—or consult the Clara Davis menu.

*More on Meat, Poultry, and Fish*

"Meat usually presents no problem to the child, a carnivorous animal," writes Helen Train Hilles in *Young Food*. "He rarely objects to juicy lamb chops, roast beef, or roast turkey." The year is 1940 and Hilles is writing for slightly older babies, but your baby is no different. Her idea of baby food is medium-rare lamb. Before I found *Young Food*, nine-month-old Julian loved to gnaw on a lamb chop.

Your baby grows on protein, iron, and zinc. Any meat, poultry, or fish will do. Liver is a time-honored first food because it's extremely high in iron. In the Siberian tundra, Nenet children eat raw liver and raw reindeer meat, often frozen. Unlike most meat, liver contains a fair amount of vitamin C, which aids iron absorption.

It's difficult to overstate the importance of iron for your growing baby. Pound for pound, his iron needs are the highest in human life. Around one year, your baby starts to run out of iron stores, and he needs to get it from food. Liver and red meat are best. Dr. Nancy Krebs, a professor of pediatrics, found that breast-fed babies who ate meat as a primary weaning food starting at four or five months grew faster than those who didn't.[4] Another study showed that adding ground meat to a typical weaning gruel made of milk and cereal increased iron absorption by 85 percent.[5] Adding vitamin C on top of that provided a dose large enough to cover iron needs in 95 percent of babies one year old.

Low iron is probably more common now because modern life is so sterile. Iron is abundant in soil. Traditionally, crawling babies and toddlers probably got a fair amount of iron from dirt floors in huts and tents.[6] Vets know that baby pigs suckled without access to soil are anemic; they fix it by putting dirt in the pen.[7] I grew up on a farm and went barefoot for ten years. I don't know how much iron you'll find in a public park or sandbox, but in the country our toddlers were frequently barefoot, if not naked, outdoors. I figure there's a lot of good stuff out there.

It's a shame that modern weaning diets call for iron-poor milk and grains. As usual, the food companies want to sell you something, and this time, it's iron-fortified baby cereal. Happily, attitudes about meat for babies are coming around again. Even the supermarket Whole Foods recommends meat as a first food, calling it "nutrient-dense," a term favored by real food folks. Whole Foods was founded by a vegetarian. The times, they are a-changin'.

Most books will tell you to purée meat in water, stock, or milk and spoon-feed your baby, which is dandy, but it seemed like a lot of work to me. Julian, Jacob, and Rose had meat on the bone or in chunks from the start. Babies tend to keep any chunks too big to swallow safely in the front in the mouth. Your baby may consider a lamb chop or drumstick a tasty teething ring. Julian loved a chicken bone.

Raw ground beef or lamb with olive oil and salt is a good dish for babies, as are sautéed ground beef and lamb, hamburger, sausages, and roast chicken or turkey. If your baby eats raw meat, make sure you trust the source. If you give her cured meats, such as salami and ham, see that they're made with real meat and don't contain junk ingredients such as nitrates and corn syrup.

Fish is also an excellent first food, any way your baby likes it. Adding a little butter will make the omega-3 fats for her brain go farther. Without a doubt, my favorite baby food was roe. Roe has it all for mother and baby. It's fun, like a bright orange pea. Your baby can pick it up, piece by sticky piece. When she bites down, it goes *pop!* It's delightfully salty, and of course it's an exemplary source of iodine and good fats. We buy frozen wild salmon roe from Alaska.

### One More Word on Iron

Rob's oldest friend, his roommate at camp and in college, is a distinguished doctor. He was an internist, trained to know something—actually quite a bit—about everything in the body of man, woman, and child. "The best doctor I ever had," says Rob. But he left medicine for the pharmaceutical business, fed up with the way things were going. "No one is properly taught in medical school anymore," he says. Beneath his executive suit still beats the heart of a medical man, a man whose job and duty are not only to diagnose and cure, but also to reassure.

How we wished he were looking after Julian! Not long after his first birthday, Julian got a virus he couldn't kick. He'd been eating plenty of real food, including meat, for a good six months, but now his appetite fell off and he nursed more. I wasn't concerned. Breast milk is best for babies whose digestion is off, and I knew he'd eat again when he was hungry. Meanwhile, he thinned out, as many babies do at this age.

At one year, our pediatrician tests every baby for iron stores, so Julian gave blood from his tiny arm. His iron and hemoglobin came back low, and the doctor prescribed inorganic iron, but I wasn't sure that was right for Julian. I suspected he was "hiding" iron from the winter viruses he kept meeting, and that absorption of all nutrients, including iron, was temporarily compromised by vomiting and diarrhea. I didn't want to make his gut flora worse with supplements. We decided to focus on iron-rich foods instead. When I declined to fill the prescription, the doctor was not pleased.

Julian kept eating red meat and liver, and at supper he had grass-fed liver in capsules. I didn't find the powdered liver too tasty, so we mixed it with maple syrup. We also limited dairy and cereals because they're iron-poor, they block iron, and they contain disaccharides, which aren't good when your gut is down. Julian kept nursing, of course, and we kept him away from the germ conventions known as baby classes. Before long, his good health, digestion, and appetite came back.

But not the iron. At the second test, his iron was up just slightly. Again the doctor urged us to give him inorganic iron, but we stuck with food. On the third test, the iron went up a little and the doctor's dander went up a lot. "If you won't give Julian *real* iron," he said, "go find another doctor."

It's not every day you get fired by the pediatrician. It was not perhaps his finest moment. But I was more puzzled than pissed off, so I kept my good humor and tried logic, even as the doctor was showing me the door. Julian was thriving, I reasoned. There was no sign of trouble with red blood cell production. He had no symptoms of anemia—from the Greek for "without blood"—such as pallor, lethargy, developmental delays, or stunted growth. On the contrary, he was energetic, cheerful—even taller. He *was* thinner than some other boys, but he ate as much real food as he wanted, including plenty of iron-rich and iron-friendly foods providing folate, vitamin $B_{12}$, and vitamin C. I knew many breast-fed babies who'd slipped under the curve on the weight chart. Finally, I mentioned my concerns about inorganic iron.

The doctor waited impatiently for me to finish. Even as I spoke, I knew there would be no exchange of ideas about iron, today or ever. Since we weren't talking about evidence-based medicine, as I understand the term, I guess the only thing Dr. Iron had left for his closing argument was exaggeration embroidered with guilt. "Julian is not growing because his red blood cells can't get any oxygen."

Maybe that works on other mothers. With me facts are more effective. When in doubt, I do homework. I asked around. "We don't test any babies for iron," said one pediatrician. "In five years of practice, I've never prescribed iron supplements to a baby and never seen anemia." "Julian probably consumes more iron than most babies in the world," said another, after taking me through an exhaustive history of Julian's health, his diet, and mine. "The problem is absorption, and supplements won't help." "The worst thing you can give a baby with diarrhea is more iron," said the expert in iron metabolism. "Inorganic iron may worsen anemia," said the gut health specialist. "The important thing about these numbers is that they're going up," said another family doctor. We gladly found another doctor. We persisted with foods, and at the next test Julian's iron levels were perfectly healthy.

Rob e-mailed his friend, the doctor, for his view. His reply to a nervous father was notable for its brevity, clinical perspective, and reassurance. "Don't all babies have low iron around twelve months?" One night at dinner, Rob asked him how he would have handled Julian's case, and he answered in a roundabout way. "We were taught that seventy percent of the diagnosis is in the patient's history and twenty percent in the physical exam. But no one even looks into the patient's eyes anymore," he lamented. "What's the other ten percent?" Rob asked. "Oh yeah," he said. "Just the tests. All these young guys do these days is send your blood off to some lab."

*More on Eggs*
Whole eggs are an excellent first food. The yolk contains several nutrients for the brain, including cholesterol, which insulates

nerve cells, omega-3 fats such as EPA and DHA, and choline. If you don't believe me, consult U.S. Patent 6149964, for a baby food recipe containing DHA-enriched egg yolks. The baby food executives aren't stupid. They'd like to sell you egg-rich baby food. You can serve eggs instead. Let the yolk be a little runny to preserve the omega-3 fats, and add a little real salt for brain cells.

Some people recommend waiting a year for egg whites because they contain hard-to-digest proteins and/or because they are allergenic. I'm not convinced on either point. The whites are, however, better when cooked. Raw egg white contains a protein called avidin, which blocks biotin, a B vitamin. According to the nutrition researcher Christopher Masterjohn, most of the avidin in a fried egg is destroyed, while gentle poaching leaves most of it intact.

Serving eggs is child's play. Kids love them. Even babies like to watch you crack them open and cook them. Our children ate them fried, sunny side up, soft-boiled, hard-boiled, and scrambled, with cheddar, Parmigiano Reggiano, salmon roe, sour cream, sautéed onions, diced tomatoes, and more besides. Boiled yolks mashed with olive oil and salt are another winning food.

### More on Milk, Cheese, and Yogurt

Rich in protein, vitamins, calcium, and good fats, dairy foods are excellent for growing babies and toddlers. Most babies make lactase to digest the lactose in cow, goat, and sheep milk, and will continue to do so as long as you give them fresh milk to drink.

Cheese, yogurt, and sour cream are cultured, which makes them even more digestible, and they're brimming with probiotics. Many babies are crazy for cheese. Julian liked the salty ones, including raw milk blue cheese. A traditional Italian baby food is grated Parmigiano Reggiano mixed with olive oil. Julian loved that, too. Today all three love cheese.

Yogurt, crème fraîche, and sour cream are tasty on all kinds of foods, from ground beef to peaches. Although you'll want to keep all sweets to a minimum, plain yogurt *is* rather sour. A wee bit of raw honey or pure maple syrup won't do any harm. Experts say that babies under one year old should not eat honey, but it seems that botulism in honey is rare.[8] Julian had a taste or two of honey before his first birthday, but it's certainly not an important first food. After one year, the one-minute dessert Julian ate most often was yogurt or crème fraîche with honey or maple syrup.

### More on Fruit and Vegetables

What a lot of hooey there is about when to give your baby certain fruits and vegetables! From what I can tell, none of it matters. I gather some parents introduce vegetables before fruits to prevent a sweet tooth, but I doubt it helps. Fears about nitrates in green vegetables are groundless. I see no reason to delay raw salad vegetables such as tomatoes or cucumbers. Your baby is not likely to be allergic to citrus. Babies have been drinking orange juice to prevent scurvy for nearly one hundred years.

I never peel fruit and vegetables, for babies or anyone else, because the vitamins and antioxidants are in and under the skin. In fruits like peaches, much of the flavor is there, too. Babies are quite competent. As soon as Julian had two front teeth, he cut right through the skin on whole nectarines by himself. If he didn't like the peel, he carefully stripped off the flesh and left it. He could hollow out grapes—a delicate operation.

You can purée raw or cooked fruit and vegetables, but I didn't bother. Right from the start, our children ate or gummed roasted zucchini chunks, tomato pieces, whole blueberries, and whole plums. They ate around peach pits. As with meat, babies tend to store larger chunks in the front of the mouth.

Fruit must be ripe. Unripe sugars will give anyone a stomachache. Tree fruits rich in pectin, such as plums, apples, and pears, may be easier for babies to digest when cooked. Homemade apple sauce is easy. Just quarter unpeeled apples and boil with a little water and a cinnamon stick until soft.

Chances are, your baby will enjoy fruit and vegetables in many sizes, shapes, and colors—or at least one or two she calls for again and again. A picky eater tends to emerge around the age of three or four, if at all. On that note, please don't start off on the wrong foot by serving the little one plain broccoli and carrots. Babies need fat, and they like salt, not to mention dill, parsley, or garlic, as much as the next guy. In our house, every man, woman, and child gets vegetables with olive oil or butter and salt. They taste better.

*More on Cereals*

You can file "Cereal Is Good" under Myths About Baby Food. Bread and porridge are poor man's baby food. The king's kids eat meat, fish, and ice cream. Grains are lousy sources of protein, iron, and zinc. They're difficult to digest, especially when they're not properly prepared. Gluten, the protein in wheat, is notably challenging to digest. The big starch-digesting enzymes don't kick in for one or two years. Until then, your baby depends on the amylase in your milk. Here is the nutritionist Jen Allbritton, whose expertise is feeding babies and kids, on cereals:

> Babies do not produce the needed enzymes to handle cereals, especially gluten-containing grains like wheat, before the age of one year. Even then, it is a common traditional practice to soak grains in water and a little yogurt or buttermilk for up to 24 hours. This process jump-starts the enzymatic activity in the food and begins breaking down some of the harder-to-digest components.

Dr. Michel Cohen is another cereal skeptic. "Years ago, eating solids early in life was considered essential," he says. "Among the principal beneficiaries of this philosophy were manufacturers of the baby cereal. Bland and slightly sweet, cereal is easily ingested by a young baby who does not need to eat solid foods yet. Nowadays, babies start on solids around six months of age, when they're ready to chew and are more coordinated, and by that point they have little interest in largely tasteless cereals." Babies "don't need cereals," says Cohen flatly. His main objections are that cereal is constipating and starchy. "An early emphasis on starch contributes to both a predilection for white foods (rice, potatoes, etc.) and the acquisition of a sweet tooth later on."

The heyday of gruel and commercial baby food is passing, and with it the cereal craze. Even Whole Foods is now a cereal skeptic. "There is no medical need to feed cereal as a first food," says the supermarket's baby food guide. Your baby does need carbohydrate, however. If she spends all her fat and protein on energy, she won't grow. Carrots, sweet potatoes, bananas, and apple sauce are good options.

It's perfectly sensible to wait a full year before offering wheat, oatmeal, or grits. Your baby won't miss anything he needs. Sensible, yes—but awfully difficult. I intended to save wheat for after Julian's first birthday, just to let his digestion mature, but some bread crept in. The best grain for babies is rice, which contains less gluten than wheat. Soak brown rice overnight, cook it well, and serve it with butter. (That said, by the age of two white rice had also passed Julian's lips.)

Oats are good, too. Around eight months Julian ate a fair number of Duchy Originals organic whole oat cakes. They were terribly handy on planes, and I reckoned they were one of the best cereals on the shelf. Then the British pound went up and up, and I couldn't justify the cost. Since then I've scoured the shops for decent crackers. Who will make a good American oat-cake with whole organic oats?

### One Word on Fats

You scarcely need to hear more from me on the subject of fats. But some mothers are afraid they will raise fat babies with heart disease by giving them real food. These fears are groundless. More than half the calories in breast milk come from fat, and more than half of that fat is saturated. It would be odd indeed if natural fats were not good for babies. The American Academy of Pediatrics agrees. "A low-fat eating plan is not advised for children under two years of age because fat is an essential nutrient that supplies energy."

### One Foolproof Food

All over the world, people consider bone broth a health tonic. In Italy, gelatin is regarded as food suitable for convalescents. Chicken soup, famously, is known as Jewish penicillin. Koreans make soups from bone marrow and guinea hen for ill and weak people. The gelatin in broth heals intestinal mucosa and cartilage reduces inflammation, which makes broth good for weak digestion and immunity.

Our nation's early champion of broth was Sally Fallon, author of the classic real food cookbook, *Nourishing Traditions*. "Although gelatin is not a complete protein, containing only the amino acids arginine and glycine in large amounts, it acts as a protein sparer, helping the poor stretch a few morsels of meat into a complete meal," she says. "During the siege of Paris, when vegetables and meat were scarce, a doctor named Guerard put his patients on gelatin bouillon with some added fat and they survived in good health." I pay attention to hardship foods because they point to what's essential.

Happiy, you can now buy good bone broth in many shops and farmers' markets. To make broth, boil bones a long time with a little acid (such as vinegar, lemon juice, or wine) to help pull the minerals out. The density of the broth indicates how much gelatin came out of the joints. When it cools, it should quiver like aspic. Skim off the fat to taste but do keep some of it. Marrow from game and grass-fed cattle contains mostly monounsaturated fat. It's also a good source of polyunsaturated fat and conjugated linoleic acid (CLA), which Loren Cordain, an expert in traditional diets, calls a "potent cancer inhibitor."[9]

Digestible, nutritious, and tasty, broth is perfect food for babies. It's good when they're thriving and when they're under the weather. Your baby can drink it from a cup or bowl. Julian's friend Huck was known to lick chicken stock off the side of the pot. You can purée meat or vegetables with broth, make gravy from it, cook rice in it, moisten yesterday's mashed potatoes with it, simmer meat or vegetables in it, and dip bread in it. You can make a terrine or just serve the gelatin. If your baby doesn't drink milk, broth is a fine source of calcium.

*A Word on Allergies*
Parents are anxious about causing allergies and food sensitivities simply by giving their babies real food. The World Health Organization, the American Academy of Pediatrics, and the European Academy of Allergology and Clinical Immunology advise avoiding solid foods for four to six months to prevent allergies later. Most advice calls for keeping your baby away from milk, wheat, eggs, citrus, soy, peanuts, and fish for a full year. Some say longer.

There is no doubt that immune-system disorders such as allergy and asthma are climbing. But is real food to blame? The most recent data undermines the conventional advice about how and when to feed your baby. In 2008, a thorough study of more than two thousand children found no evidence that delaying the introduction of solid foods past four or six months prevents asthma, or allergies to food, pollen, or pets at six years.[10] The researchers tested milk, wheat, eggs, soy, rye, peanuts, and fish.

Some experts are concerned about the trend for "nut-free" spaces. Writing in the 2008 *British Medical Journal*, Harvard professor and physician Nicholas A. Christakis says that nut bans are counterproductive. The bans are an overreaction to the size of the threat, not proven to be effective, and will increase sensitivity to nuts due to lack of exposure. "The cycle of increasing anxiety, draconian measures, and increasing nut allergies must be broken."

Your baby is not likely to have a serious food allergy or intolerance. About one baby in a hundred is allergic to peanuts. Less than 1 percent of children cannot digest gluten. About 150 people of all ages die each year from food allergies. If your baby does react to a food, you're almost certain to notice symptoms right away. Bad reactions to milk and peanuts tend to show up early. Bad reactions to eggs tend to occur later, well after first foods. Fish allergy is just plain rare in babies.

Julian, Jacob, and Rose ate all the alleged allergens (except soy) long before turning one. They ate fish, shellfish, citrus, eggs, cow milk, wheat, rye, and every nut I can think of, including peanuts. The only foods we avoided are the industrial foods we don't eat anyway, such as corn and soybean oil and industrial soy protein, which is a common allergen.

Allergies, eczema, food sensitivities, and digestive disturbances, from malabsorption to irritable bowel syndrome, have many known causes and still more undiscovered ones. We cannot address them properly here, but I'm happy to suggest an ounce of prevention. Breast-feed your baby. (The National Institute of Allergy and Infectious Diseases recommends strict breast-feeding for at least six months.) Keep nursing well after your baby starts eating. Delay or space vaccinations. Feed your baby all the known allergens within twelve months. Spend time on farms, touching animals and dirt, and drink raw milk.[11] The human gut and immune system appear to prefer exposure for proper development.

## THE SCIENTIFIC FEEDING METHOD

Now that your baby is ready—and I'm assuming you're ready, too—it's time to eat. These are my highly technical, thoroughly researched instructions.

Put some real food in front of your baby. Keep him company while he touches it, moves it around, stacks it up, rubs it in his elbow, and pokes it between your lips. If any of it reaches his, don't shout, do a fist bump, call his father, call your shrink, or even comment. Now wash anything or anyone sticky. Do the same thing, once or twice a day—maybe when you eat, if that suits you—for the next few weeks or months.

That's all. I didn't buy baby food or make it. I didn't mill or purée anything. Sometimes Julian nursed before a meal, sometimes after. I didn't buy any new ingredients. I didn't buy special dishes with compartments. Five months after he started eating, someone gave him plates and utensils. (What's less useful than a baby knife?) Until then he used his hands. Sometime after that, I realized that he loved tiny spoons and bowls, so I found cheap ones in Chinatown.

Julian had his first proper meal around seven months. It broke all the rules. It contained three or four ingredients, not one. It included three alleged allergens: cow milk, citrus, and eggs. It even broke my own rule, in that he had a little sugar. He ate a lightly cooked egg yolk with a bit of unrefined sea salt. He had two lightly sweetened yogurts, orange and lemon. Our friend Patrick Lango, a chef and dairy farmer, makes them from his own grass-fed milk. Patrick's White Cow Dairy recipes, including his unsurpassed custard and yogurt cream, are the only foods Julian has eaten from a jar.

Some people recommend feeding your baby in stages: first by spoon, then giving finger foods, and finally letting the baby use utensils. All I see in this advice is more work for mothers. In *The Family Book of Child Care*, Niles Newton says a five-month-old can feed himself. "He may enjoy putting gobs of cottage cheese, scrambled eggs, or thick cereal into his mouth . . . solid items like cheese or meat can be cut into long thin pieces about the size of half a pencil. Babies like to work their strong jaw on such solid substances even though little may be swallowed."

Two weeks after his first meal of yogurt and eggs, Julian and I were well into our own self-selection diet experiment, with one glaring difference. My method was somewhat sloppier than the Clara Davis approach. I did it the easy way.

> New foods these last ten days: guacamole (previously only plain avocado); cayenne pepper; olive oil and virgin coconut oil on my nipples . . . more White Cow Dairy yogurt and custard; more crème fraîche; sucking on a piece of chicken; more egg; salsa on an egg; a dark black cherry; a strawberry; white peaches; yellow nectarines; apple; chèvre on cucumber; banana-milk-coconut pudding with cinnamon and cayenne; olive oil and avocado dressing; banana with crème fraîche, coconut, and cinnamon.

Three days later, more firsts. "Finely grated Parmigiano Reggiano with olive oil, which he actually seemed to love, organic roast chicken drumstick; chicken soup; some blue cheese, some 85% Lindt chocolate, a grape or two, strawberries." I gave Julian whatever I was eating and didn't worry. If he had a bad reaction to something, we'd figure it out.

Perhaps you have higher standards. In baby matters, I start with the minimalist position and only concede the activities or purchases I consider absolutely necessary or highly entertaining. We have been more successful in some spheres than others. As a baby, Julian owned too many stuffed animals (all gifts) but never too many trucks. We tried cloth diapers, but within days, I knew chlorine-free disposables were for us. We try to make up for this ecological sin by putting poop in the potty, where it belongs. Accordingly, at two years old Julian owned—and used—six potties.

When it was time for Julian to eat, I had not forgotten the Eden of nursing. So tidy. So little effort for me. I made precious few concessions on new ingredients and preparation methods. I can think of a hundred activities I prefer to making baby food. I did start buying two things—grapes and frozen peas—from the supermarket, because they're handy, he loves them, and so do I. Reluctantly, I found we could not manage without decent crackers.

We did concede valuable freezer space to two items just for Julian. One day, I was baking sweet potatoes and had too many, so I stuck raw slices in the freezer. If there are no leftover vegetables, Judy, his nanny, can pull spuds from the freezer for Julian's lunch. In minutes they're boiled and buttered. Julian often eats leftover meat, but I found it convenient to freeze little lumps of ground beef, lamb, and pork. With this small effort, there's always a Julian-sized portion of meat handy.

With one two-year-old the scorecard on baby clutter in our small kitchen didn't look too bad. New items: peas, grapes, and (mostly) whole grain crackers. New chores: freeze sweet potatoes and meat. New stuff: one chair, two bibs, tiny spoons, and a half dozen little wooden bowls. I felt good about the paraphernalia level.

For lazy mothers like me, the good news is that feeding your baby what you're eating is the best way to feed your baby. There is every reason for your baby to eat your Bolognese sauce or roasted vegetables. You can mash it up with a fork if you want, but there's no need to pulverize it. Giving your baby your dinner will be faster than making a separate dish and cheaper and better than any baby food you buy.

Once you put food in front of him, try to let the baby choose what he wants. Easier said than done, I know. Don't micromanage meals. Don't point things out and pick things up. Don't stare at him. Offer more only when he runs out. If he declines one thing or another, by all means try again another day, but not every day for a month. Julian ate apples twice. Then politely ignored them. For a while I offered apples, and then I stopped. He didn't like mashed potatoes or homemade applesauce.

Try to show no reaction, good or bad, to what your baby eats. Not so easy, either—but worth it. At six months, when you've just begun, this is merely good policy. It's essential later, if your baby is a birdlike or selective eater. Train yourself not to comment now, and it will be easier not to comment later, when it matters more. I'm dwelling on this good advice because with Julian I found it so hard to follow. It got easier with Rose and Jacob.

*Pablum* is the commercial name of an early baby food, invented in 1930 and sold by Mead Johnson. Now it has come to mean bland pulp or worthless ideas. Your baby deserves better than bland. Show a little respect for her palate and present a range of flavors, including sour, salty, spicy, and bitter. Julian got dark chocolate from the beginning; bitter is what chocolate means to him. He liked salty cheese and coffee-spiked milk.

A restaurant critic told me she started her six-month-old on cereal, as the doctor recommended. The baby was bored and constipated. When her mother liberated herself—and make no mistake, it's not only the baby who's trapped by such rules—the baby rejoiced, asking for banana, avocado, and gorditas, lime-soaked corn tortillas topped with spicy meat.

On a warm night in Seattle, Julian and I were having dinner after a book event and chatting with an Indian woman about the word "heat." "People assume 'spicy' means hot," she said. "But many of our dishes, while richly spiced, are mild." When you feed your baby, consider all the spices in your pantry. Cinnamon, for example, is wonderful on mashed banana with milk or coconut cream. I read somewhere that Ayurvedic principles call for "warming" milk, which is considered "cool," with cinnamon, but that's not why I do it. I'm crazy about cinnamon, and when Julian seemed to like it, I put it on everything. Feeding your baby is very scientific, you see.

## BABY DRINKS

The best drinks for your baby are pure water and real milk. For at least six months, breast milk can quench her thirst even as it fills her belly. But breast milk is quite sweet, and as she grows, she'll sometimes want water only. I remember hot summer days when Julian refused warm breast milk in favor of cold water.

Timing is not important. You can offer milk and water whenever you start offering food. If you start food later—at seven or eight or nine months—there's no harm in offering water sooner, around six months. When you have a babysitter or need to leave longer stretches between nursings, it's nice if your baby is willing and able to have a sip of water. Having a word or sign for water is great. If the baby is fussy merely because she's thirsty, she can say so.

Milk is the other best drink for babies. It is both food and drink, of course, and that's a big reason it's so valuable. Precious few liquids contain protein, calcium, vitamins, and good fats. Perhaps more to the point, most kids love it. Milk is the rare traditional food that never fell out of favor with baby experts. You can introduce milk whenever you start offering food.

The American Academy of Pediatrics says that babies up to two years old need whole milk, not skim. But I think everyone is better off drinking whole milk. I also suspect the two-year cut-off is arbitrary. A three-year-old, of course, is still growing. Why would skim milk suddenly be better for him? Whole milk contains fat-soluble vitamins, readily available calcium, and glycosphingolipids, special fats that protect against intestinal infection.

Julian loved dairy of all kinds, but he didn't come to like milk until he was well past a year. It didn't matter, except that I had always imagined Julian clutching a cup of raw grass-fed milk, the best food in the world. As I keep learning, a mother's expectations are so hard to avoid, so seldom useful.

One Wednesday in August 2007, the *New York Times* sealed Julian's reputation as a milk drinker with an enormous photo of Rob, Julian, and me, with a sippy cup of raw milk looming in the foreground. The headline asked, SHOULD THIS MILK BE LEGAL? The reporter Joe Drape had decided Julian was the news. "Nina

Planck, the author of *Real Food: What to Eat and Why*, defied the FDA's warning and drank raw milk while she was pregnant," he wrote. "She not only continues to drink it while nursing her 9-month-old son, Julian, but also allows him the occasional sip."

We had a good time reading the letters. To my surprise, there was only one nasty one, from an overheated Washington lawyer comparing my behavior to "wanton and reckless child abuse." Other voices spoke up for objective standards in food safety, informed choice, nutrition, flavor. "You are the poster girl for Hot Mama Eats Right and Has Fun," wrote Anne Watkins. "But that crazy headline—why not, 'Should So Many Lousy, Sloppy and Wrong-Headed Regulations by the FDA Be Legal?'"

For several weeks, messages blew in from Rob's childhood crowd in Highland Park, New Jersey. "We knew you had a cheese shop," they said. "But we didn't know you were nuts." Needless to say, Rob and I think the world's gone mad, not us. I grew up on raw milk. As for Rob, after thirty years in the grocery business, he has boarded more than a few flights from Paris with raw milk cheese stashed in his carry-on. A veteran of food fights, he is always on the side of flavor and tradition.

I did feel guilty about one thing. Try as I might, I wasn't able to tap into the local black market for real food that summer. We were renting a house in East Hampton. We had no trouble buying local corn and peaches, but in that zip code, the people eating steamed fish and vegetables still outnumber the ones who eat lard. To supply the photographer with the image he required, I had to order the grass-fed milk from Organic Pastures, a dairy near Fresno, California.

Julian did drink milk that summer, including raw milk, just not very much. He preferred peaches and bananas mashed with Organic Pastures raw cream. In September, we headed back to the city, and I went back to work in my little office across the street. Once Julian was settled with his new nanny, I confess that I did try to encourage milk drinking. It's such a healthy snack.

I tried a few things with our little milk-skeptic. I added a dash of local juice—usually raspberry or tart cherry—which makes a thin, pink, yogurtlike drink, more tart than sweet. We called it a milk shake, and he liked it. I also made cinnamon milk and chocolate milk with unsweetened cocoa powder. He loved both. Whether these concoctions made a whit of difference I'll never know, but eventually he was a regular milk drinker. As a toddler, he would set out with his nanny and two no-spill cups, one for milk, the other for water. I approve of raw milk, but we mostly drink pasteurized milk.

If someone suspects your baby is not eating enough, milk may be an issue. Some experts will tell you to limit milk because babies fill up on it at the expense of other good food. Just as many experts advise giving milk at meals and between them to increase nutrients and calories. Some of my friends offer only water with meals, so the children do not fill up on milk at the expense of dinner. There is no right answer. When Julian was on the slim side and the pediatrician was giving us a handout titled "Increasing Calories in Your Child's Diet," I considered his milk consumption—cow and breast—carefully. There was nary a sign that milk affected his appetite either way.

If yours is the rare baby with a confirmed allergy to milk casein, don't worry. *Just don't give your baby milk.* Find the nutrients in milk in other foods, such as chicken soup. I don't recommend imitation milks made with soy, rice, or almonds. They don't provide the same nutrients as milk, and they often contain vegetable oils, thickening agents, and sugar.

A hundred years ago, babies used to get a little fresh orange juice to prevent scurvy. Now scurvy is rare. There's plenty of vitamin C in the produce section of the sorriest supermarket. Sometime between then and now, drinking juice got out of hand. Babies drink apple juice in bottles and sippy cups, while toddlers are always clutching those little boxes with straws.

This is bad news. Sweet and filling, juice displaces more nutritious foods. For thirst, water is better. For vitamin C, potassium, and antioxidants, fruit is better. Most juice is pasteurized, which reduces its vitamin C content. For vitamins A and D and calcium, milk is better. Juice contains no fiber to cushion the blood sugar and slow the insulin spike.

An early juice habit may be bad news later. Researchers at Deakin University in Melbourne found children aged four to twelve who had about two glasses of fruit juice or juice drink per day were more likely to be overweight or obese.[12] The more juice, the greater the risk of being fat. We've seen similar trends in the United States and Britain.

That said, I've let Julian take glugs of tart cherry juice straight from the bottle in the fridge. It's quite sharp, but it's juice. He had more than one sip of orange juice before he turned one. And once, at a street fair on a very hot day, I was happy to share my smoothie made with whole fruit and lots of pineapple juice with Julian. It was terribly sweet, and we both enjoyed it enormously. (I'm forced to tell you such things. If I don't, someone will spot me and ruin my reputation.) All of our children drink some juice, mostly local cider or raw orange juice.

Bottles and cups are indispensable equipment. What kind of cup is up to you and your baby. We tried a regular bottle a couple of times, and a soft, breast-shaped bottle called Adiri, but Julian wasn't keen. He never used a nipple. When he started to drink milk and water around seven months, he used our cups and glasses, with help. Later I bought a no-spill cup for outings. Stainless steel and glass are the best materials.

We made very little effort with vessels, largely because I dislike baby gear. At home and at our Waldorf School, our children used small glass tumblers even as toddlers. Some will master bottles, spill-proof cups, and real cups sooner, some later. It simply doesn't matter how or when your baby drinks from a cup, as long as your baby gets enough to drink.

## I GET IN HOT WATER OVER VEGAN BABIES

Crown Shakur was six weeks old and weighed three and a half pounds when he died. His vegan mother and father, who fed him mostly apple juice and soy milk, were convicted of murder and cruelty. It was the third such conviction of vegan parents in several years. My heart went out to Crown's parents, and the others, too. They belong in school, not in jail. It's scary that anyone might think soy milk could keep a baby alive.

After I blogged on vegan diets for babies, the *New York Times* asked me to write something about feeding infants for the op-ed page. The day before my piece ran, I spoke to the editor. "We have a great illustration," he said, "I think you'll like it."

It was my fifth piece for the paper, but I'm always a little jumpy the night before publication. On May 21, 2007, I got up early to look for my op-ed online. The editor was right. The commissioned illustration, by Jacob Magraw-Mickelson, was great. It depicted a mobile, the kind you hang over a crib. Dangling from it were fish and salad leaves. Clever.

I didn't rest my eyes on the sketch for long. When I saw the headline, my heart sank. DEATH BY VEGANISM. I'd written that poor Crown died of ignorance, not veganism. I would have used different words in the headline. But that wasn't going to matter to vegan parents.

My op-ed was the most e-mailed item on the *New York Times* Web site. According to the paper's ombudsman, Clark Hoyt, the "torrent" of letters was still flowing two months later. He decided to examine the editors' decision to run the piece. When he tracked me down in a hotel in San Francisco, his first question—"Are you aware that the American Dietetic Association (now the Academy of Nutrition and Dietetics) says that a well-planned vegan diet is appropriate for pregnancy, nursing, and infancy?"—had that *gotcha!* quality. "Yes, I am," I answered. "I don't agree." There was a brief silence while he pondered his next question. In the end, Hoyt concluded that the editors were entitled to present my point of view. "Planck has her experts," he said.

The evidence for vegan diets in infancy and childhood presented in the Academy paper is weak or absent. But the authors are quite clear on one point. "The safety of extremely restrictive diets such as fruitarian and raw foods diets has not been studied in children. These diets can be very low in energy, protein, some vitamins, and some minerals and cannot be recommended for infants and children." The authors do not explain how a diet exclusively of plants differs from the "extremely restrictive diets" mentioned above. Elsewhere, however, they note that "little information about the growth of nonmacrobiotic vegan children has been published," and once again recommend supplements for vegan babies, children, and teens.

When Julian and I got home, exhilarated and exhausted after a week of book signings in San Francisco, Portland, Seattle, and the San Juan Islands, Rob gave me a tight hug. I slept a long time. The next day, we all piled on the Hampton Jitney and headed back to the house we'd rented for the summer. I was glad to be lying low in the woods. I've had stalkers, threats, and hateful letters before.

For a couple of weeks, I ignored strange names in my in box. If the subject line was suggestive—say, "Your Vileness"—I left the e-mail unopened. But eventually, I read every one. A few were thoughtful, intelligent, and polite. Conscientious parents told me about feeding their vegan babies with great care. I used to be a careful vegan, so I know what it takes to eat well. I admire their commitment and effort, and we can agree that industrial farming is shameful.

More than a year later, I've examined every issue again, from vitamin $B_{12}$ to DHA. This debate comes down to one thing: reproduction. An otherwise healthy adult may follow a vegan diet and do fine for a while, perhaps even for his whole life. But in traditional societies, the vegan diet is unheard of. It's just not good enough for babies and children. "When women avoid all animal foods, their babies are born small, they grow very slowly, and they are developmentally retarded," says Lindsay Allen, director of the U.S. Human Nutrition Research Center. "It's unethical for parents to bring up their children as strict vegans."[13]

Vegan parents are correct that breast milk is best. But as we've seen, vegan breast milk lacks vital DHA. In vegan communities strictly opposed to taking supplements, mother's milk is low in protein, carbohydrate, and total fat. The babies in these communities, who are weaned on soy, suffer from growth retardation, protein and calorie malnutrition, iron- and $B_{12}$-deficiency anemia, rickets, zinc deficiency, and chronic infections.[14] Soy is a poor source of iron, calcium, and zinc. It lacks adequate methionine, which babies need to grow, and damages the thyroid, which hinders immunity and stunts growth.

The greatest growth spurt in human life takes place between late pregnancy and age two, and the brain is highly vulnerable to malnutrition until age three. Babies who are ready to leave the breast behind need protein, omega-3 fats, iron, calcium, and zinc. Compared with meat, fish, eggs, and milk, plants are inferior sources of every one. In "Nutrition, Growth, and Complementary Feeding of the Breastfed Infant," Kathryn Dewey writes, "Predominantly vegetarian diets cannot meet nutrient needs of breastfed infants unless nutrient supplements or fortified products are used."

Last but not least, malnutrition is cumulative. Key nutrients lacking on a vegan diet, such as vitamin $B_{12}$ and DHA, are depleted with each pregnancy and each generation. That's why you don't find generations of vegans in traditional groups. I was pondering these matters when the following letter arrived from Amber Hill, in Grass Valley, California.

I am mother to Mycelia, born two months before your Julian. I had a mostly vegan pregnancy and early postpartum period, and did pretty well for a while. But by six months I was exhausted, weak, depleted, and too thin. I thought of life with my baby more as a game of survival than anything else. Many people had mentioned traditional foods, and after much persuasion on my part, my husband Graham Hayes, a fabulous chef trained in the vegan tradition, and I started to eat in a whole new way. I'm sure you know the rest—I feel a million times better than I have in years, my daughter is a plump, happy, and very healthy eighteen-month-old now, and we started a business delivering nutrient-dense foods and teaching classes to prenatal and postpartum moms! Thank you Nina, so very much, for facilitating a profound shift in the life of my family, and for providing me a resource to point to when telling people about good food!

—Amber

P.S. Are you writing a book called *Real Baby Food*?

It was nice to hear from sunny Amber in darkest February. I was spending too much time at my desk. I desperately wanted some sun, but that would have to wait. Meanwhile, I was hungry for a hot meal, one I hadn't cooked. Thinking other working mothers might feel the same—I mean tired and hungry—I started a list on my Web site, REAL FOOD DELIVERED, to spread the word about similar businesses (although Amber's has since closed). This book is dedicated to Amber and her family, and to everyone who feeds mothers and babies.

## BREAD AND CHOCOLATE

We had friends over for brunch. I put out what Rob would call "a nice spread." There were bagels and all kinds of breads, there was wild cured salmon, wild smoked sable fish, scrambled eggs with butter and milk, plenty of good cream cheese, a large green salad. Julian, now a toddler, had a plate full of good food before him, but he hadn't started on the fish and eggs yet. He was too busy braying for bread. It was difficult to ignore. "Can he have some?" said my friends. "No," I said. I told Julian, who was sitting next to me with an imploring expression, the same. A few minutes later, a hungry boy was digging into fish and eggs. I found myself relieved—the bread battle was over, for the moment—but also self-conscious.

My two friends at brunch that day had seven children between them. These children eat white flour, and they are visibly strong, healthy, and intelligent. "There isn't a total white-flour ban, I just want you to know," I said, unprompted. "It's just that when he fills up on bread first, he doesn't eat anything else. I mean, it's not my goal that Julian never eats any bread or junk food, ever." They read my tone correctly: I was afraid of looking like a loony and creating a taboo so great Julian would do anything to get his hands on white bread when I'm not looking. They smiled sweetly and said, "We don't think you're crazy, Nina."

In fact Julian had eaten his share of white bread and crackers, despite my no-Goldfish, no-Cheerios policy or, more precisely, hopes. My first goal is good ingredients. We prefer to give him unsweetened whole grains, such as whole oat crackers. But in practice he's had plenty of Duchy Originals oat cakes sweetened with a little Demerara sugar and plenty of cheese crackers made with white flour, cheddar, and butter—especially on the road. I look for whole grains, traditional fats, and minimal added sweeteners. That's my idea of decent baked goods for meals and snacks, but we also eat white sourdough and Pullman loaves. It is difficult to feed a child beef stew and raw milk on airplanes. Hats off to mothers who carry grass-fed beef jerky and goodness knows what else.

My second goal was to let our children know, over time, why we favor certain foods over others. Proper bread made from white flour is not pure junk food, but it's not great food, either. The nutritional value of any bread, white or whole grain, is improved by schmeering it with butter, almond butter, or olive oil, or by dunking it in milk or beef stock or chicken soup. When our kids are in a bread and cracker mood, we do all these things.

My third goal is not to let them fill up on baked goods before eating fat and protein. There is a place for baked goods.

Babies and children need ample carbohydrate as well as protein and fat; otherwise they would spend the protein and fat on energy and have nothing to grow on. In modern life, it's difficult—though possible, if you insisted on it—to give a toddler all his starches from cooked vegetables and fruits. I don't try. My main goal is nutrient-dense foods, and white bread isn't one. It's nutrient-poor—and filling. After they eat some combination of meat, fish, dairy, fats, fruits, and vegetables, we serve bread, and after that, sometimes a real dessert.

If there lives a mother who can keep her little sweetie innocent of sugar for longer than a year, hats off to her. I don't mean the fructose in whole fruit, or even a little honey or maple syrup, but white sugar. It's everywhere. We were quite strict about sugar, but I didn't try to ban it. When ours started eating, each got a little dark chocolate from time to time. Julian ate his first proper dessert—a classic cheesecake from Murray's Cheese—on his first birthday. As he got older, he ate dark chocolate and ice cream more often.

Dessert appears under certain conditions. It comes in small portions, after meals, and on special occasions. Dessert is real food, which means it contains good ingredients, like cream. It's not too sweet. I hope that tolerating a few good sweets in moderation will serve us later, when they are old enough to get their hands on sugar independently. I found validation for this approach from Helen Train Hilles, in *Young Food*.

It is expedient to take the lure out of candy by making it legal. You don't want to put your child in the position of having to outwit you. He's going to eat candy anyway, and you can really decide only whether he shall do it with your sanction or on the sly. If he does it on the sly, as any intelligent child who is denied all freedom will, you bring upon yourself far more serious problems than the effect of a couple of jaw-breakers on his system.

I thought things were going pretty well. Julian was about sixteen months old. He ate a lot of real food, and I wasn't too neurotic about the treats. Then Julian "fell off" the weight chart, and Dr. Iron got that stern look. "He needs to stop nursing, and he needs to eat more calories." I was confused and said so. This was a boy who sat down for three meals daily. He got red meat daily, he'd never seen a vegetable without olive oil, and he was welcome to good bread with butter. His latest dessert was crème fraîche with honey and nuts. As for nursing, I'd seen him nurse before big meals and after them. I didn't see any sign that nursing affected his appetite. So what if he was thinner than most babies his age? Most breast-fed babies are. "Someone has to be off the weight charts," I said. The doctor looked like thunder, but I wasn't trying to be funny. I was trying to be logical. Most babies are in the middle of the curve, but some mother's baby has to be at either end, right?

Dr. Iron, never one for dialogue, didn't even address this point. His instructions were clear: Julian must stop nursing, and he must eat more. He sent me home with a list of caloric foods: whole milk, cheese, ice cream, butter, milk shakes, almond butter, eggs, bacon, sausage, guacamole. We were only to steer clear of juice, white rice, and pasta.

Nothing wrong with the foods. Just that I wasn't worried about Julian's growth, size, or weight, any more than I was worried about his iron. His head kept expanding. He was two inches taller and two pounds heavier since the last visit. He was physically active, sociable, a great talker. His joints were plump with what they call growth fat. He'd done what many babies do around age one. They grow up and stretch out, like hand-pulled mozzarella.

At home, I looked at the handouts. *Your Growing Child: Eighteen to Twenty-Four Months.* Everything it said described Julian: "Has about twelve teeth." Check. "Sleeps ten to twelve hours." Check. "Walks up stairs without help." Check. "Weighs twenty to twenty-eight pounds." Check. (On *this* chart, his weight was within "normal.") On language, habits, affection, the pamphlet described Julian to a tee. "No!" is probably becoming a familiar expression, it said. You bet it was.

Next I read about feeding. "Growth slows down abruptly after the first year and appetite decreases. A child who ate hungrily several months ago will now sit and pick at food," said the handout, quoting the pediatrician Barton Schmitt, author of *Your Child's Health*. I read the symptoms.

> It seems to you that your child doesn't eat enough.
> Your child's energy level remains normal.
> Your child is growing normally.
> Your child is between one and five years old.

That was Julian—except that only Dr. Iron thought he wasn't eating enough. I laughed out loud at the last line. For these *four* years parents drive themselves crazy worrying about calories, weight, and growth? I wasn't laughing when I came to the diagnosis. The heading was "Appetite Slump in Toddlers," but the technical term for this condition is "physiological anorexia." Why do doctors make a pathology out of a developmental stage even they acknowledge is normal? More to the point, did Dr. Iron read his own handouts?

Of course it didn't matter if Julian weighed twenty-one pounds and other toddlers weighed twenty-eight. But my conversation with the doctor had made me nervous about Julian's weight, so I cut back on nursing and tried to make him eat more. He seemed only to eat less. Worse, he demanded more bread, crackers, and chocolate. Now, in addition to worrying that he was too thin, I was mortified. I had raised my very own monovore. *Julian will gain weight on this plan*, I thought bitterly—*and be diabetic*.

Clara Davis haunted me. I was supposed to stay neutral, to show no reaction. But privately I was praying, cheering, despairing over one spoonful or another. I got mad when Julian left good food uneaten or threw it on the floor. When I gave him sautéed ground lamb and buttered sweet potatoes, peas with olive oil, and or crème fraîche with honey and coconut—things he once loved—and he asked for crackers, I felt like crying.

I did cry. I cried privately, I cried in front of Rob, and I cried on the phone to my mother. Once I got mad and tried to feed Julian with a spoon. We had never spoon-fed him. That made him cry, and that made me cry. These are not my proudest moments.

Everyone could see that I needed to back off. Even his mother finally got the message. "Don't hover over your baby's every bite," Niles Newton wrote in 1957. "Don't talk to him or distract him, or give him so much food or so many eating utensils that he can make very complicated games out of his food. Never comment on what he is eating or not eating. Never urge him to eat. Simply remove the food when he dawdles." Dr. Schmitt had similar advice.

Put your child in charge of what he eats.
Never feed your child if she can feed herself.
Offer finger foods.
Serve small portions.
Avoid talk of eating.
Don't extend mealtimes.

Notice what they don't say. "Try to make your child eat more." All this advice boils down to one thing: Do less.

It's hard to avoid getting emotionally involved in your child's nutrition. It's not a logical thing to ask of a mother. *Of course you're emotionally involved.* You're in charge of this little creature. You fed him with your own body. Just try to keep your head on straight. Try to be concerned without being anxious, alert without being hypervigilant, informed without being a slave to facts.

When at last I did relax, things got better immediately. I don't mean Julian ate more. Sometimes he ate more, sometimes less. I mean that my relationship with Julian got better—dramatically better. He stopped begging for bread and chocolate. And he grew like a weed.

## COD LIVER OIL COMES BACK

*I want my cod liver oil and I want it now.*
—Woody Guthrie, *Songs to Grow on for Mother and Child*

Woody Guthrie wrote many songs for the kids in his life and recorded two wonderful records for Folkways in 1956. When I was little, the car song was a great favorite in our house, and little Julian loved it too. By quoting this verse, I don't mean to suggest that 1940s and 1950s babies were lining up demanding cod liver oil. Cod liver oil is not delicious. I mention it only to illustrate that cod liver oil was once considered a terrific food for small children.

In 1940, Helen Train Hilles published *Young Food*, a practical guide to feeding children. Vitamins and their functions were just being discovered, nutrition was becoming (apparently) more scientific, doctors were in charge of dinner, and mothers were as worried about whether their babies got enough of these magical, mysterious and invisible ingredients as we are about omega-3 fats.

> We are pathetically anxious to be good mothers . . . We worry about such things as vitamins; yet they have existed for more years than we have known about them. It is hard to avoid them. They lurk in unexpected quarters and may even be found in potato skins . . . Maybe we don't need to worry quite as much as we do; maybe we rely too much on rules and terms and not enough on our own common sense.

The author was not under the spell of nutritionism. "We are almost convinced that without cod liver oil the baby would get rickets," she wrote, exasperated by the worry spilling over every dinner table. Her message is simple. Real food will do for the whole family.

Yet Dr. J. Taylor Howell, a "leading New York pediatrician," was apparently compelled, in the Age of Vitamins, to conclude his foreword to her book this way:

> In this book the subject of vitamins has not been discussed, for in many instances the rapidly changing knowledge in this field makes it difficult to be too dogmatic about their full value at the present time. The foods in a well-planned diet contain many of the vitamins that are essential to the growth and well-being of the child, but as this cannot be depended upon at all times, I would be remiss if I did not call attention to the importance of the proper use of cod liver oil, or its equivalent, and orange juice to fortify the daily diet.

Mothers and doctors alike knew that cod liver oil would prevent rickets and orange juice would prevent scurvy. Hilles, a mother, was right to focus on food, not on vitamins. The doctor, who had no doubt seen his share of malnutrition, was right to mention the best way to improve a poor diet. If only mothers and doctors today were as sensible.

Vitamin A, usually in the form of fish liver oil (cod or halibut) or butter, has a long history as a supplement for babies and children.[15] In the 1920s, nurses in maternity wards, hospitals, and orphanages routinely gave cod liver oil to their charges. During the Second World War, the British Ministry of Food provided cod liver oil for pregnant and nursing women and children under five. Throughout the twentieth century, nannies and mothers gave American and European children cod liver oil and orange juice each morning.

Much of the prewar research on vitamin A concerned infectious diseases. Vitamin A looked promising for prevention of measles and other infections. In the 1920s and 1930s, pharmaceutical companies aggressively promoted cod liver oil. A Squibb ad warned that whooping cough, measles, mumps, chicken pox, and scarlet fever "may do greater harm than most mothers think." But children would have lighter cases, recover faster, and be less likely to suffer "permanent injury" if they built up "resistance" with cod liver oil.

In the 1940s, the arrival and spread of powerful antibiotics, so effective at treating infectious diseases, choked off research in vitamin A as the "anti-infective therapy." Sigh. Another dead end for nutritional research. But I don't let the history of food and medicine get me down. Pharmaceutical companies, once enthusiastic, are through with cod liver oil? Fine. We'll look after our health in the traditional way—with food—and use supplements and medicine when we need it.

At about one year, Julian started taking a teaspoon of cod liver oil and grass-fed butter oil every day, or most days, anyway. It's the classic nutrient-dense food. A 1930s ad for Parke-Davis cod liver oil boasted that one teaspoon provided the equivalent quantity of vitamin A in five and one half quarts of milk, nine eggs, or one pound of "best creamery butter."

In addition to vitamins A and D, cod liver oil is a modest source of omega-3 fats. If you add grass-fed butter oil, or just serve plenty of butter, your baby will get plenty of vitamin $K_2$, a great combination for healthy bones and teeth. Babies with dark skin and those who don't get enough direct sunlight will benefit even more. During the coldest six months of the year, Nebraskans need an extra 1,000 IU of vitamin D to reach optimal blood levels for calcium absorption.[16]

Julian never enjoyed drinking his cod liver oil—not even Cinnamon Tingle—but I was willing to make him, on most days, anyway, because I believed in it. It protected him from the vagaries of weaning diets and the viral assaults of toddlerhood. He usually enjoyed a small square of dark chocolate after glugging it down. Liquid cod liver is messy, too. Later, I gave all three children chewable cod liver oil, and after that I mostly stopped. They're pretty well-fed, and I don't want any of us taking too many supplements for too long.


## BYE BYE, DELICIOUS MILK

Watching older babies nurse makes some people uncomfortable. Don't let that stop you. People have all kinds of ideas about nursing. ("When he can ask for it, it's time to stop.") Having teeth or being able to walk, talk, and eat solid food are not markers for weaning. None of these milestones has any clinical or nutritional relevance.

It's all up to you and your baby. Though it's uncommon today, there is nothing unnatural about nursing longer than the full year the American Academy of Pediatrics recommends. The AAP recommends nursing as long as mother and baby desire, and the World Health Organization says "two years and beyond" is good.

All the benefits of your milk—nutritional and immune-related—continue as long as your baby drinks it. In the second year, your milk contains a surprising amount of protein, vitamins, and minerals, and a higher percentage of fat.[17] Your milk is simply more concentrated, which makes it even better food than ever. Rather like cod liver oil, breast milk enhances the uneven toddler diet.

Julian was like many babies and toddlers, in his love for nursing beyond hunger and thirst. Any nursing mother knows how handy it can be after a scare, a scrape, or a shot. The comforts of nursing are one of its sweeter benefits.

Perhaps your child will ease off slowly, nursing less and less, or perhaps you will have to stop cold turkey for some reason. Some people say that "child-led" weaning is a myth, but that's too strong. I guess it's true, if you mean that toddlers don't wake up one day and announce, "Thank you for the breast milk. I'm big now and I've had enough." No, they seldom do that. But many babies do participate in saying good-bye to the breast.

## NURSING YOUR TODDLER

In the second year, 450 milliliters (15 ounces) of breast milk provides the following nutrients.

| NUTRIENTS | PERCENTAGE IN MILK |
|---|---|
| Energy | 29 |
| Protein | 43 |
| Calcium | 36 |
| Vitamin A | 75 |
| Folate | 76 |
| Vitamin B$_{12}$ | 94 |
| Vitamin C | 60 |

SOURCE: K.G. Dewey, "Nutrition, Growth, and Complementary Feeding of the Breastfed Infant," *Pediatric Clinics of North America* 48, no. 1 (February 2001).

Because there is no medical need to wean or proven superior approach, no one can tell you when or how to do it. This is the time to get inspiration and comfort from other mothers and to listen for what might suit you.

At one year, I gradually weaned Julian for work (mine) and sleep (mine). I didn't try to do it quickly, because I found it stressful for both of us. In a couple of months, he didn't nurse at night, and he didn't nurse from nine A.M. to six P.M. on weekdays. He kept nursing each morning and evening on weekdays, and on weekends and holidays.

At about nineteen months, I held back the breast on the days we spent together. Julian was furious. He pestered me constantly for "baba" and nursed more than ever when he got it at night. It was very tiring for us, and after weeks of struggle, I decided we weren't ready. When I let him nurse again by day, he asked for it less.

A few months later, when Julian was two years old, we decided to have another baby, so it was time for me to wean him. He had shown no signs of stopping, or slowing down in any way, so I stopped letting him nurse on a Friday. We had a trying weekend in the country. On Monday morning, I told his nanny. Julian, overhearing me, looked up from his breakfast, and said, "Mama baba *all* done?" His eyes were wide. I felt terrible.

Other babies I knew were more apt to let it go. Sara weaned Ursula overnight at fifteen months. Two weeks later, Ursula had a cold, and Sara offered her the breast. Ursula swatted it away, as you would a pesky fly. The advantages of turning off the spigot just like that are clear. It's quick and simple.

One thing is sure. Every mother tells me that the right time to wean is when *you* are ready to wean. "You have to know that it's what you want and be strong about it," said my friend Indya. "We wanted to have another baby, so my motives were clear." Nursing, especially night-nursing, reduces fertility. If you aren't happy nursing your toddler, that's enough reason to stop. When you do stop, be clear in your own mind that it's time, clear about why, and clear with your nursling. Your toddler deserves an explanation—not a dissertation, just a nice, clear message—and a consistent policy.

For Rose and Jacob I wanted to do it differently. Highly social children with big and diverse appetites, they were very different from their big brother, so I had little trepidation about weaning, but I wanted to mark the occasion. I want to teach my children how to honor milestones and to say good-bye. (Even adults need more practice with endings.) On Valentine's Day, we invited family and friends to a Bye Bye Baba party. Rose and Jacob were two-and-a-half. We served lunch. For dessert I made "baba cakes": four-inch cheesecakes. We decorated the apartment with red paper hearts and huge two-breasted helium balloons. Julian, Jacob, and Rose each got a soft toy breast, the kind you find in adult stores. Pinkish, plump, and satisfyingly squishy, they were the hit of the party. In a few weeks, they shriveled up and were forgotten. (Just like real breasts, I thought.) My friend Indya wrote and recorded a song called "Bye Bye Babas." We must have played it in the car a hundred times.

> Now it's time to say bye to babas
> Now we can hug and kiss and snuggle with Mommy
> And drink cow's milk
> But still it's hard to say bye to babas
> Bye bye babas

When you wean, be kind to yourself as well as your baby. In the days and weeks after the last nursing, you may feel sad because a uniquely sweet activity is passing. As prolactin levels fall, you may also feel tearful for physiological reasons. This is common, normal, and temporary.

Babies do remember nursing. In *Fresh Milk: The Secret Life of Breasts*, Fiona Giles collected memories from young children. An older sister who had been weaned acted out her own farewell as she watched the new baby nurse. She covered her mother's breasts and said, "Bye bye, delicious milk."

## THE STATE OF REAL FOOD, CIRCA 1940

On May 1, 2008, Rob and I bought a country place in Stockton, New Jersey, thirty-seven acres of woods and pasture with an old stone house built around 1768. We call it Small Farm, after Farmer Small in the Lois Lenski book *The Little Farm*. One hot weekend in July, there was plenty of action at Small Farm. Julian was going on two and just hitting his stride. Having thought a long time about walking, he now seemed to find it useful, and he talked a blue streak. (On the potty: "Come, pee!")

We visited Oscar, the German shepherd puppy next door. When Julian saw two rows of nipples on Oscar's mother, he correctly identified her as the source of the puppy's "baba." We chased frogs in the pool and picked wineberries in a thunderstorm. But in those days, nothing rivaled digger action. When our neighbor brought his dump truck, brush hog, and tree chipper to mow the pastures and take out dead trees, Julian was literally panting with pleasure.

The pasture hadn't been mowed all year, so there was enough hay to bale, but on Small Farm our projects are Small and Smaller. Instead of hiring a baler, we set out with the wheelbarrow, and a nineteenth-century rake we found on the farm. Julian and I quickly filled the wheelbarrow with hot, dry grass. He wanted to push it, but it was too tall, so he settled for riding home atop our little haystack, rake teetering.

That summer Small Farm had one crop: tomatoes. Two tomatoes, actually—one Sun Gold and one Cherokee Purple. My parents brought them from Virginia. Each week, Julian and I watered the tomatoes, adding a spoonful of Growers, a natural mineral fertilizer, to the watering can. Each week for three weeks, he had carefully picked and eaten one tiny ripe golden cherry tomato. "More?" he asked, signing with his hands at the same time. Alas, no. We mulched our tiny crop and put the rest of the hay in the shed, although I doubted we'd find anything else to do with it.

Later that day, we were browsing in antique shops in Lambertville, a small town just down the Delaware River. A lot of kid stuff was better back then, so I had to restrain myself. Julian already had two vintage wagons from my mother. He had a chalkboard made of real slate and an elegant folding wooden lawn chair, to mention just two finds from local flea markets. An old-time red Tonka pickup was tempting, but Julian had lots of trucks, and it cost forty dollars. But when we saw the little blue and red wheelbarrow minutes later, we had to take it home. I figured Farmer Small needed a few tools his own size.

In the same shop, Rob spotted *Young Food*. In 1940, it sold for $2.50, but we were glad to pay ten dollars. Once I read it, I knew I would've paid fifty. It was the best book on feeding real food to the whole family I'd ever seen. My heart swelled as I read how Helen Train Hilles described life before the war. You could buy raw milk. Milk meant whole milk, of course. The "druggist" sold ice cream cones, and you can bet they weren't made from soy protein. Lamb chops and egg custard, not juice boxes and fish-shaped crackers, were considered foolproof foods for children.

It all sounded so traditional. And yet, in 1940, Hilles already believed that modern life was sweeping away the best American foodways. I smiled, but felt bittersweet, when I read the heading of the final chapter, "A Plea for Tradition in Food."

> Whatever you do, if your child is a city child, don't let him miss the priceless joy of country meals, even if you have to beg, borrow, or steal a country relative. A farm is ideal. No egg will ever taste as good as the one gathered (with some trepidation on account of the fluttering hen) warm from the nest and carried carefully home in cupped palm; the still warm tomato plucked from a vine so pungent that it almost makes you feel dizzy; the slightly fuzzy taste of New Zealand spinach broken, a leaf or two at will, from quickly multiplying leaves; radishes and onions, carrots and beets, pulled tiny and crisp and earthy from the yielding earth; tender young broilers—unless he has made a pet of them and knows them by name, for even without feathers, old Joe will not make enjoyable eating for any child—butter fresh from the churn he has helped to turn; the long cooling drink of buttermilk; fresh milk, or cream from the tops of the pans laid out in the heavenly cool of the cellar or well-house; a tall crunchy stalk of rhubarb, chewed for its juices and then discarded.

Maybe we'll never get around to my dream of buying a cow—someone has to milk her, and it won't be Rob—but we love the frog pond, the woods, and the meadows, and we can manage a few crops. Fortunately, we can buy all manner of real food at Stockton Market, the tiny Sergeantsville farmers' market on Saturdays, and at the bigger Sunday market, farther down the road at the old Dvoor dairy place. Small Farm may never produce the truckloads of vegetables of my childhood, but the day came when we picked figs, herbs, cherry tomatoes, and flowers, and we all love our small flock of summer chickens. In the meantime, for Julian, Rose, and Jacob, I'm sure that a very small farm is better than no farm at all.

# Afterword: Only Her Mother

*Experience: that most brutal of teachers. But you learn, my God do you learn.*

—C. S. Lewis

Motherhood has taught me to prefer experience to other forms of knowledge acquisition, such as books, folk wisdom, mother's advice, and expert opinion. A lifelong fan of facts, logic, and analysis, along with my old friend homework, I was astonished (and eventually pleased) to discover this. Book learning has often failed me, either because memory fails or because what I have read could not outlast my own stubborn opinions. A mother's advice is priceless, of course, as anyone who has grown up without a mother knows, and yet . . . it's only one woman's opinion. Folk wisdom may endure, but it's not always accurate; lore is best paired with objective data. Experts, meanwhile, may lack feeling; they think in terms of populations, not persons.

But my own lived experience, what a trove! It's free, hard to ignore, and impossible to forget. Oddly enough, time and memory seem to work in my favor. In other words, after a disagreeable experience, the pain fades in time, but the lesson sticks. My pleasant memories fade quickly too, so it seems I need to acquire new pleasant experiences on a regular basis. Joy-amnesia becomes a fine reason to seek the fun in life, over and over again.

When I finished writing *Real Food for Mother and Baby*, Julian was two years old. A few months later I was pregnant with twins. Eight years later, my thoughts on mothering are different, partly because Jacob and Rose are not Julian, and partly because I have changed. In this new edition, I've updated facts where they've changed, but in the foregoing pages I've preserved my state of mind, circa 2008, on pregnancy, childbirth, breastfeeding, and the feeding of young children.

I will not be the first to say that being a wife and mother is humbling. This was driven home to me when Rose was five months old. A tiny but springy thing, she had just begun to pull herself up to standing. I sat on the couch, watching her balance on two feet, holding a toy. She dropped the toy. She looked at me; she looked at the toy. She whimpered for the toy. I watched her. It would have been easy to pick up the toy, but I didn't. She whined some more. At last, after what seemed like an age to me, tiny Rose slowly, carefully, bent her knees, and, balancing herself with one hand on my knee, squatted to grab the toy. She straightened up and held it aloft. Rose was triumphant. I was crying. "I am only her mother," I thought. I was overwhelmed by the minor role I was playing. It seemed to me that the best thing I could do for Rose was to stay out of her way.

Let your baby do what she can do—no more and no less. This is anathema to helicopter parents. I learned not to cajole, entertain, or "help," my babies from Resources for Infant Educarers (RIE), an awkward name for a genius organization based on the pioneering work of a Jewish Hungarian pediatrician called Emmi Pikler, who founded the Lóczy orphanage in 1946 and ran it until 1979. Pikler and her followers show us how to step back so our babies can do more. After RIE training (it is definitely training), you will never again be able to tolerate the ceaseless exhortations of modern ambitious parents. "Look at the birdy! Clap! Catch the ball! Where is the dog? Walk to Daddy! Who is that? What's her name? You remember Uncle Billy! Look who's getting tired! Who's feeling a bit shy today?" Between all the questions, answers, directions, and questionable labeling of subjective, private mood states, the poor infant, toddler, or primary schooler hasn't a chance to think, feel, move, or speak for himself. To be "only" their mother: this is how I interpret humility. I frequently fail, of course.

Rose and Jacob also taught me that your next baby will not be like the last one. I knew this in theory, of course. Even when we treat them the same, children are vastly different. My blissful pregnancy with Julian was followed by a tricky labor. Weaning was sad. While pregnant with Rose and Jacob, I was anxious, heavy, out of breath, off-balance, and tired. For the first three months, we fretted about unexplained bleeding, and until the very end I was throwing up. But their birth was a breeze. Even though I had pre-eclampsia at thirty-eight weeks and was, at thirty-eight years old, of "advanced maternal age," I had a VBAC—no, *two* VBACS. Breastfeeding and weaning were easy.

The differences persist, maybe even deepen, with age. When we had three children under three, I kept overstating my influence and forgetting how different they were. One is a beautiful sleeper who would, even as a tiny baby, turn away from a cuddle when it was time to cross the threshold. Another didn't sleep through the night until miraculous tonsil surgery. At six years old, the third was still waking up frequently. One quit night-time diapers at two and a half years and woke up dry every morning. Another finished bed wetting three years later. One is a true omnivore. Always hungry, the child has never missed a nursing, meal, or a snack. Another is a selective eater and a separatist (foods must not touch) with the sensitive palate of a supertaster. Most of these differences, I am convinced, are temperamental and innate, immune to the environment of our home. Some reflect the normal range of development, others special needs.

One of our children had trouble falling asleep, napped poorly, and woke frequently. I finally realized that the problem was not pathological. Once I accepted the reality, I was able to see the solution: throw more human labor at the problem, in the form of my body or that of another family companion. But before that, when the child was one or two, I lamented my broken sleep with a mother whose child slept beautifully. "Well, you see," she said earnestly, "I put a lot of time and effort into good sleep habits." At that moment I realized that mothers innocently overstate their role. I'm sure she did put effort into healthy sleep, but so had I, and two of mine slept well. The child who always wants to be held, the lousy sleeper, the bed-wetter, the mitten-loser, the finicky eater . . . the parents of these children put far more time and effort into "good" habits than the parents of children who come to these things easily. After hearing the unconscious bias of maternal agency in her voice, I was less judgmental, of others and myself.

When Rose and Jacob were one year old and Julian was nearly four, Rob and I got married at Small Farm. Motherhood and marriage have taught me the value of service. For my enlightened friends, service is not an appealing term. But I don't see it that way. It's my daily practice, and my calling, to serve the needs of our family, including my own. To serve each of us properly often requires me to sacrifice something. If service were cost-free, would it be service? I have found it easier to submit to the task, to go about it with a cheerful purpose, than to resist it. Submission and sacrifice are strong, perhaps even offensive terms, to modern women; maybe "surrender" is better. In any case your gift must be freely given.

However you characterize your role, I think it's false to suggest that being a good wife and a good mother can be achieved while pursuing one's own will at all times. Don't misunderstand. I have not stopped nourishing myself. I have learned to do less of what doesn't matter, and more of what does; I seek help from my husband, children, family, and friends; and I care for myself better than in my twenties and thirties. If you do not already have a regular physical practice, a faithful social net, and a spiritual life, motherhood is a good reason to pursue all three.

How, exactly, to serve each child is trickier. After the child's needs for food, shelter, and love are met, each of us benefits from slightly different medicine: more discipline here, more empathy there. In any realm—sleep, clothing, nutrition, physical development, social life—my aim is to serve the person before me, given his or her biological and temperamental capacity and limits. There is no point in forcing my son to wear wool if it's unbearably scratchy, no point in asking my husband to enjoy a piece of chewy beef (even if it is grass-fed), and no point in suppressing the irrational exuberance and mysterious melancholy in our high-volume, passionate family. If anything has changed since 2008, it's the slow erosion of my obstinacy. Although we live within a framework of inherited and chosen values (good food, individual freedom, joint responsibility, family loyalty) the more I say yes to my husband and children, the more fun we have.

Sometimes I play a parlor game called "No One Told Me." We all heard stories before becoming mothers. What *didn't* you hear? What would you like to pass on? This is how I answer. Being a mother and wife is a magnificent experience, often intensely joyful. At the same time, being a good mother and a good wife is extremely difficult. Just how difficult, however, I wouldn't want to learn from a book.

# Appreciation

Without my agent, Jennifer Unter, there would be no book in your hands. Elizabeth Tarpy provided platinum research, and Kathy Belden, my much-missed editor at Bloomsbury, made astute suggestions. For this spectacular tenth-anniversary edition, I am in debt to my editors Rachel Mannheimer and Laura Phillips, and to Patti Ratchford and Katya Mezhibovskaya, who designed the beautiful new cover. I am grateful to the marvelous Martha Wilkie for her work on this book (and others) and for her friendship. I thank the many readers who have written to me about *Real Food for Mother and Baby* and spread its gospel. Finally, I would like to thank my mother, for her birth and my birth.

# Notes

## CHAPTER 1: WHAT IS REAL FOOD?

1   B. Lata and K. Tomala, "Apple Peel as a Contributor to Whole Fruit Quantity of Potentially Healthful Bioactive Compounds. Cultivar and Year Implication," *Journal of Agricultural and Food Chemistry* 55, no. 26 (December 2007): 10795–802.

2   David R. Jacobs Jr. and Linda C. Tapsell, "Food, Not Nutrients, Is the Fundamental Unit in Nutrition," *Nutrition Reviews* 65, no. 10 (2007): 439–50.

3   R. A. Fielda et al., "Iron, Zinc and Alpha-Tocopherol Content of Bovine Hemopoietic Marrow," *Journal of Food Composition and Analysis* 15, no. 1 (February 2002): 19–25.

4   Essential reading for the problems with the lipid hypothesis. Uffe Ravnskov, *The Cholesterol Myths: Exposing the Fallacy That Saturated Fat and Cholesterol Cause Heart Disease*; Gary Taubes, *Good Calories, Bad Calories: Challenging the Conventional Wisdom on Diet, Weight Control, and Disease*; and Kilmer S. McCully and Martha McCully, *The Heart Revolution: The Extraordinary Discovery That Finally Laid the Cholesterol Myth to Rest and Put Good Food Back on the Table*.

5   F. B. Hu, M. J. Stampfer, et al., "A Prospective Study of Egg Consumption and Risk of Cardiovascular Disease in Men and Women," *Journal of the American Medical Association* 281, no. 15 (1999): 1387–94.

6   International Coenzyme $Q_{10}$ Association to U.S. Food and Drug Administration, September 5, 2001. The International Coenzyme $Q_{10}$ Association, a body of scientists and medical professionals who conduct extensive research on coenzyme $Q_{10}$, issued a letter to the FDA, noting that statins block the biosynthesis of coenzyme $Q_{10}$. Ironically, coenzyme $Q_{10}$ is critical for proper

heart function, and the letter states that "although statin therapy has been shown to have benefits, the long-term response in ischemic heart disease may have been blunted due to the $CoQ_{10}$ depleting effect" and cites several sources.

7    Martha M. Kramer, F. Latzke, and M. M. Shaw, "A Comparison of Raw, Pasteurized, Evaporated and Dried Milks as Sources of Calcium and Phosphorus for the Human Subject," *Journal of Biological Chemistry* 79 (1928): 283–95.

8    For more on the nutritional changes when milk is ultrapasteurized, see: R. P. W. Williams, "The Relationship Between the Composition of Milk and the Properties of Bulk Milk Properties," *Australian Journal of Dairy Technology* 57, no. 1 (April 2002): 30–44; and Nivedita Datta, Hilton C. Deeth, et al., "Ultra-high-temperature (UHT) Treatment of Milk: Comparison of Direct and Indirect Modes of Heating," *Australian Journal of Dairy Technology* 57, no. 3 (October 2002): 211–27.

9    Richard E. McDonald and David B. Min, eds., *Food Lipids and Health* (New York: Marcel Dekker, 1996). This volume is part of the Institute of Food Technologists Basic Symposium Series. See the chapter "Food Lipids and Bone Health" by Bruce A. Watkins and Mark F. Seifert, 98–101.

10   S. H. Swan et al., "Semen Quality of Fertile U.S. Males in Relation to Their Mothers' Beef Consumption During Pregnancy," *Journal of Human Reproduction* 22, no. 6 (2007): 1497–1502.

11   Gary Taubes, *Good Calories, Bad Calories: Challenging the Conventional Wisdom on Diet, Weight Control, and Disease* (New York: Alfred A. Knopf, 2007), 232–33.

12   Food and Nutrition Board, Institute of Medicine of the National Academies, National Academy of Sciences, "Letter Report on Dietary Reference Intakes for Trans Fatty Acids. Drawn from the report on Dietary Reference Intakes for Energy, Carbohydrate, Fiber, Fat, Fatty Acids, Cholesterol, Protein, and Amino Acids," 2002, 4, 14.

13   Kalyana Sundram, Tilakavati Karupaiah, and K. C. Hayes, "Stearic Acid-Rich Interesterified Fat and Trans-Rich Fat Raise the LDL/HDL Ratio and Plasma Glucose Relative to Palm Olein in Humans," *Nutrition and Metabolism* 4 (January 2007). Accessed online at http://www.nutritionandmetabolism.com/content/4/1/3.

14   David R. Jacobs Jr. and Linda C. Tapsell, "Food, Not Nutrients, Is the Fundamental Unit in Nutrition," *Nutrition Reviews* 65, no. 10 (2007): 439–50.

## CHAPTER 2: THE FERTILITY DIET

1 Courtney Van de Weyer et al., *Changing Diets, Changing Minds: How Food Affects Mental Well-Being and Behavior* (Winter 2005), 21.

2 Two pioneers discovered and disseminated evidence for the fetal origins of adult conditions. In the late 1980s, the late Dr. David Barker published several now-famous papers showing a link between newborn and adult health. The other is French obstetrician Dr. Michel Odent. Search his database for links between the perinatal period (conception to one year) and adult health at www.primalhealthresearch.com, or for an introduction to his work, read *Primal Health*.

3 R. A. Waterland and R. L. Jirtle, "Early Nutrition, Epigenetic Changes at Transposons and Imprinted Genes, and Enhanced Susceptibility to Adult Chronic Diseases," *Nutrition* 20 (2004): 63–86. S. A. Ross, "Diet and DNA Methylation Interactions in Cancer Prevention," *Annals of the New York Academy of Sciences* 983 (2003): 197–207.

4 R. A. Waterland and R. L. Jirtle, "Transposable Elements: Targets for Early Nutritional Effects on Epigenetic Gene Regulation," *Molecular and Cellular Biology* 23 (2003): 5293–300.

5 Read and search the entire book at http://gutenberg.net.au/ebooks02/0200251h.html.

6 Chris Masterjohn, "Vitamins for Fetal Development: Conception to Birth," *Wise Traditions in Food, Farming, and the Healing Arts* (the journal of the Weston A. Price Foundation) 8, no. 4 (Winter 2007): 24–35.

7 M. W. Pascal, "Marginal Maternal Vitamin $B_{12}$ Status Increases the Risk of Offspring with Spina Bifida," *American Journal of Obstetrics and Gynecology* 191, no. 1 (2004): 11–17.

8 Chavarro, Willett, and Skerrett, *Fertility Diet*, 134.

9 B. C. Davis and P. M. Kris-Etherton, "Achieving Optimal Essential Fatty Acid Status in Vegetarians: Current Knowledge and Practical Implications," *American Journal of Clinical Nutrition* 78, no. 3 (2003): 640S–646S.

10 Eaton et al., *Paleolithic Prescription*, 95.

11 Berger, Goldstein, and Fuerst, *The Couple's Guide to Fertility*, 41–42.

12 Y. Ishizuki, Y. Hirooka, Y. Murata, and K. Togashi, "The Effects on the Thyroid Gland of Soybeans Administered Experimentally

in Healthy Subjects," *Nippon Naibunpi Gakkai Zasshi* 67, no. 5 (May 1991): 622–29.

13    Daniel, *The Whole Soy Story*, 359.

14    The FDA specialists are D. M. Sheehan and D. R. Doerge, and the quote is from a letter that included pages of citations supporting their view. (Dockets Management Branch [HFA-305], Food and Drug Administration, February 18, 1999.)

15    Melody J. Brown et al., "Carotenoid Bioavailability Is Higher from Salads Ingested with Full-fat than with Fat-reduced Salad Dressings as Measured with Electrochemical Detection," *American Journal of Clinical Nutrition* 80, no. 2 (August 2004): 396–403.

16    Groll and Groll, *Fertility Foods*, 188.

17    Chavarro, Willett, and Skerrett, *Fertility Diet*, 51.

18    Quoted in Singer, *Garden of Fertility*, 181. See also Thomas S. Cowan with Sally Fallon and Jaimen McMillan, *The Fourfold Path to Healing: Working with the Laws of Nutrition, Therapeutics, Movement and Meditation in the Art of Medicine* (Washington, D.C.: New Trends, 2004), or www.FourFoldHealing.com.

19    Chavarro, Willett, and Skerrett, *Fertility Diet*, 124–26.

20    Ibid., 123.

21    Ibid., 143.

22    X. Weng, R. Odouli, and D.-K. Li, "Maternal Caffeine Consumption During Pregnancy and the Risk of Miscarriage: A Prospective Cohort Study," *American Journal of Obstetrics and Gynecology*, first published online in January 2008.

23    Chavarro, Willett, and Skerrett, *Fertility Diet*, 148–51.

24    Singer, *Garden of Fertility*, 167.

25    Mary Enig's comments on this paper (M. H. Zile, "Function of Vitamin A in Vertebrate Embryologic Development," *Journal of Nutrition* 131 [2001]: 705–8) can be found at www.westonaprice .org/knowyourfats/vitamin-a-fetal.html. Accessed January 21, 2008.

26    Singer, *Garden of Fertility*, 170.

27    M. F. Holick, "Vitamin D Deficiency," *New England Journal of Medicine* 357, no. 3 (July 2007): 266–81.

28    P. Mastroiacovo et al., "High Vitamin A Intake in Early Pregnancy and Major Malformations: A Multicenter Prospective Controlled Study," *Teratology* 59, no. 1, 7–11. Published online, January 28, 1999.

29  Christopher Masterjohn, "On the Trail of the Elusive X-Factor: A Sixty-Two-Year-Old Mystery Finally Solved," *Wise Traditions in Food, Farming, and the Healing Arts* 8, no. 1 (Spring 2007): 14–32.

30  C. S. Yajnik et al., "Vitamin $B_{12}$ and Folate Concentrations During Pregnancy and Insulin Resistance in the Offspring: The Pune Maternal Nutrition Study," *Diabetologia* 51, no. 1 (January 2008): 29–38.

31  Masterjohn, "Vitamins for Fetal Development," 32.

32  G. M. Shaw et al., "Periconceptional Dietary Intake of Choline and Betaine and Neural Tube Defects in Offspring," *American Journal of Epidemiology* 160 (2004): 102–9.

33  Masterjohn, "Vitamins for Fetal Development," 32.

34  Elizabeth Carlsen et al., "Evidence for Decreasing Quality of Semen During the Past 50 Years," *British Medical Journal* 305 (1992): 609–13.

35  S. Sanjose, E. Roman, and V. Beral, "Low Birthweight and Pre-term Delivery, Scotland, 1981–1984: Effects of Parents' Occupation," *Lancet* 338 (1991): 428.

36  J. Kline, Z. Stein, M. Hatch, et al., *Surveillance of Parental Employment and Spontaneous Abortion.* Final report to the National Institute for Occupational Safety and Health, Cincinnati, Ohio, 1982.

37  L. M. Frazier, "Reproductive Disorders Associated with Pesticide Exposure," *Journal of Agromedic*ine 12, no. 1 (2007): 27–37.

38  E. Tielemans et al., "Pesticide Exposure and Decreased Fertilization Rates *in Vitro*," *Lancet* 254 (August 1999): 484–85.

39  V. F. Garry, "Birth Defects, Season of Conception, and Sex of Children Born to Pesticide Applicators Living in the Red River Valley of Minnesota, USA," *Environmental Health Perspectives* 110, Suppl 3 (June 2002): 441–49.

40  K. D. Mattix, "Incidence of Abdominal Wall Defects Is Related to Surface Water Atrazine and Nitrate Levels," *Journal of Pediatric Surgery* 42, no. 6 (June 2007): 947–49.

41  F. H. Pierik et al., "Maternal and Paternal Risk Factors for Cryptorchidism and Hypospadias: A Case-Control Study in Newborn Boys," *Environmental Health Perspectives* 112 (2004): 1570–76.

42  Odent, *Farmer and Obstetrician*, 14–15.

43  W. Y. Wong, H. M. Merkus, C. M. Thomas, et al., "Effects of Folic Acid and Zinc Sulfate on Male Factor Subfertility: A

Double-Blind, Randomized, Placebo-Controlled Trial," *Fertility and Sterility* 77 (2002): 491–98.

44   S. S. Young et al., "The Association of Folate, Zinc, and Antioxidant Intake with Sperm Aneuploidy in Healthy Non-Smoking Men," *Human Reproduction*, March 20, 2008, 1–9.

45   Daniel, *The Whole Soy Story*, 368.

46   Jorge Chavarro et al., "Soy Food and Isoflavone Intake in Relation to Semen Quality Parameters." Chavarro presented this research at the 2007 conference of the American Society of Reproductive Medicine.

47   Chavarro, Willett, and Skerrett, *Fertility Diet*, 190.

48   Michel Odent, "Womb Ecology: New Reasons and New Ways to Prepare the Prenatal Environment," *Primal Health Research* 13, no. 2 (Autumn 2005): 1–7.

## CHAPTER 3: FORTY WEEKS

1   K. Räikkönen. "Sweet Babies: Chocolate Consumption During Pregnancy and Infant Temperament at Six Months," *Early Human Development* 76, no. 2 (2004): 139–45.

2   Maija H. Zile, "Function of Vitamin A in Vertebrate Embryonic Development," *Journal of Nutrition* 131 (2001): 705–8.

3   A. S. Olafsdottir et al., "Relationship Between Dietary Intake of Cod Liver Oil in Early Pregnancy and Birthweight," *British Journal of Obstetrics and Gynecology* 112, no. 4 (April 2005): 424–29.

4   Report from the Select Committee on "Inquiry into Drunkenness," House of Commons Library, August 5, 1834.

5   Eaton et al., *Paleolithic Prescription*, 61.

6   Courtney Van de Weyer et al., *Changing Diets, Changing Minds: How Food Affects Mental Well-Being and Behavior* (Winter 2005), 22. This report can be purchased from SUSTAIN: The Alliance for Better Food and Farming at www.SustainWeb.org.

7   Steingraber, *Having Faith*, 19.

8   Kaledin, *Morning Sickness Companion*, 65–66.

9   Steingraber, *Having Faith*, 22–23.

10   J. W. Sparks and L. Cetin, "Determinants of Fetal Growth, in *Neonatal Nutrition and Metabolism*, ed. P. J. Thureen and W. W. Hay, 2nd. ed. (Cambridge, Mass.: Cambridge University Press, 2006), 26.

11  See, for example, M. E. Cogswell et al., "Iron Supplementation During Pregnancy, Anemia, and Birth Weight: A Randomized Controlled Trial," *American Journal of Clinical Nutrition* 78, no. 4 (October 2003): 773–81 and the accompanying editorial, Kathleen M. Rasmussen and Rebecca J. Stoltzfus, "Editorial: New Evidence That Iron Supplementation During Pregnancy Improves Birth Weight: New Scientific Questions," ibid., 673–74.

12  B. S. Alper et al., "Using Ferritin Levels to Determine Iron-Deficiency Anemia in Pregnancy," *Journal of Family Practice* 49 (2000): 829–32.

13  Odent, *Farmer and Obstetrician*, 132–33.

14  Smith, *Infant Survival Guide*, 80.

15  Odent, *Cesarean*, 116.

16  Campbell-McBride, *Gut and Psychology*, 23.

17  E. D. Weinberg, "Iron Withholding: A Defense Against Viral Infections," *Biometals* 9, no. 4 (October 1996): 393–99.

18  M. Makrides, J. Hawkes, M. Neumann, et al., "Nutritional Effect of Including Egg Yolk in the Weaning Diet of Breast-fed and Formula-fed Infants: A Randomized Controlled Trial," *American Journal of Clinical Nutrition* 75 (June 2002): 1084–92.

19  Sussi B. Baech et al., "Nonheme-iron Absorption from a Phytate-rich Meal Is Increased by the Addition of Small Amounts of Pork Meat," *American Journal of Clinical Nutrition* 77, no. 1 (January 2003): 173–79.

20  M. Sebold et al., "Scientific Report of a Clinical Trial to Assess the Actual Absorption and Utilization of the Iron Compound Present in the Preparation of Floradix," First Medical Clinic of University of Munich, 1964.

21  Brewer and Brewer, *What Every Pregnant Woman Should Know*, 23.

22  Odent, *Cesarean*, 116.

23  Harper, *Gentle Birth Choices*, 55.

24  Harper, Ibid., 55.

25  Odent, *Primal Health*, 23.

26  Ibid. 48.

27  W. D. Rees, F. A. Wilson, and C. A. Maloney, "Sulfur Amino Acid Metabolism in Pregnancy: The Impact of Methionine in the Maternal Diet," *Journal of Nutrition* 136, Suppl. 6 (2006): 1701S–1705S.

28    Daniel, *The Whole Soy Story*, 373.

29    Rebecca DerSimonian and Richard J. Levine, "Resolving
      Discrepancies Between a Meta-analysis and a Subsequent Large
      Controlled Trial," *Journal of the American Medical Association*
      282 (1999): 664–70.

30    Patrick H. Torney, "Prolonged, On-Demand Breast-feeding and
      Dental Decay: An Investigation," M. Dent. Science thesis,
      Dublin, Ireland, October 1992.

31    Rose, *Rebuild from Depression*, 80.

32    American Academy of Pediatrics, Committee on Nutrition, "The
      Prophylactic Requirement and Toxicity of Vitamin D," *Pediatrics*
      31, no. 3 (March 1963): 512–25.

33    Van de Weyer et al., "Changing Diets, Changing Minds," 23.

34    *DHASCO and ARASCO Oils as Sources of Long-Chain Polyun-
      saturated Fatty Acids in Infant Formula: A Safety Assessment,"*
      Technical Report Series No. 22, Food Standards Australia New
      Zealand, June 2003.

35    Van de Weyer et al., "Changing Diets, Changing Minds," 24.

36    Michel Odent, "Mercury Exposure During the Primal Period,"
      *Journal of Prenatal and Perinatal Psychology and Health* 18, no. 3
      (Spring 2004): 212–20.

37    "Study Finds Government Advisories on Fish Consumption and
      Mercury May Do More Harm than Good," press release,
      Harvard School of Public Health, October 19, 2005. See also
      Eric Nagourney, "Public Health: Before Avoiding Fish, a Word
      to the Wise," *New York Times*, October 25, 2005.

38    Joseph R. Hibbeln et al., "Maternal Seafood Consumption in
      Pregnancy and Neurodevelopmental Outcomes in Childhood
      (ALSPAC study): An Observational Cohort Study," *Lancet* 369,
      no. 9561 (February 2007): 578–85.

39    Gary J. Myers et al., "Prenatal Methylmercury Exposure from Ocean
      Fish Consumption in the Seychelles Child Development Study,"
      *Lancet* 361, no. 9370 (May 2003): 1686–92. See also the accompanying
      editorial: Constantine G. Lyketsos, "Should Pregnant Women Avoid
      Eating Fish? Lessons from the Seychelles," ibid., 1667–68.

40    Harper, *Gentle Birth Choices*, 67.

41    Goer, *Thinking Woman's Guide*, 55.

42    Nancy Griffin, "Let the Baby Decide: The Case Against Induc-
      ing Labor," *Mothering*, March–April 2001. Accessed online at
      http://mothering.com/articles/pregnancy_birth/birth_preparation/
      inducing.html.

43 D. Briscoe et al., "Management of Pregnancy Beyond Forty Weeks' Gestation," *American Family Physician* 71, no. 10 (May 2005): 1935.
44 Ibid.
45 Griffin, "Let the Baby Decide."
46 Kitzinger, *Complete Book of Pregnancy and Childbirth*, 241.
47 Ibid., 346.
48 H. Akinbi et al., "Host Defense Proteins in Vernix Caseosa and Amniotic Fluid," *American Journal of Obstetrics and Gynecology* 191, no. 6 (2004): 2090–96.
49 Baumslag and Michels, *Milk, Money, and Madness*, 86.
50 A. M. Molloy et al., "Choline and Homocysteine Interrelations in Umbilical Cord and Maternal Plasma at Delivery," *American Journal of Clinical Nutrition* 82, no. 4 (October 2005): 836–42.
51 A. Kariminia et al., "Randomised Controlled Trial of Effect of Hands and Knees Posturing on Incidence of Occiput Posterior Position at Birth," *British Medical Journal* 328 (7438): 490.
52 Michel Odent, "Occiput Posterior Position Should Be Exceptionally Rare at Birth," *Midwifery Today*, Winter 2005, 22.
53 Harper, *Gentle Birth Choices*, 74.
54 Buckley, *Gentle Birth*, 131.
55 Harper, *Gentle Birth Choices*, 72.
56 Ibid.
57 Michael Odent's databank, www.PrimalHealthResearch.com.

## CHAPTER 4: NURSING YOUR BABY
1 Mohrbacher and Kendall-Tacket, *Breastfeeding Made Simple*, 6.
2 Steingraber, *Having Faith*, 238–39.
3 P. Hegardt et al., "Amylase in Milk from Mothers of Preterm and Term Infants," *Journal of Pediatric Gastroenterology and Nutrition* 3 (1984): 563–66.
4 Mohrbacher and Kendall-Tacket, *Breastfeeding Made Simple*, 5.
5 SIDS is not really a diagnosis in that it's only used when the cause of death is unknown. Sleeping with your baby can prevent SIDS if, and only if, you are not obese or drunk. Fumes from toxic bedding may be one reason babies stop breathing. For this interesting but still controversial theory, see *The Cot Death Cover-Up?* by the New Zealand forensic researcher Jim Sprott.

6   H. Kimata, "Laughter Elevates the Levels of Breast-milk
    Melatonin," *Journal of Psychosomatic Research* 62, no. 6 (June
    2007): 699–702. Available online May 30, 2007.

7   J. Menella and G. Beauchamp, "The Effects of Repeated
    Exposure to Garlic-Flavored Milk on the Nursling's Behavior,"
    *Pediatric Research* 34 (1993): 805–8.

8   "Prevention of Rickets and Vitamin D Deficiency: New Guide-
    lines for Vitamin D Intake," American Academy of Pediatricians
    Clinical Report, *Pediatrics* 111, no. 4 (April 2003): 908–10.

9   A. S. Olafsdottir et al., "Fat-soluble Vitamins in the Maternal
    Diet, Influence of Cod Liver Oil Supplementation and Impact of
    the Maternal Diet on Human Milk Composition," *Annals of
    Nutrition and Metabolism* 45, no. 6 (2001): 265–72.

10  *DHASCO and ARASCO Oils as Sources of Long-Chain Polyun-
    saturated Fatty Acids in Infant Formula: A Safety Assessment,*
    Technical Report Series No. 22, Food Standards Australia New
    Zealand, June 2003.

11  Odent, *Farmer and Obstetrician*, 10–11.

12  Read all about it (in French) at www.membres.lycos.fr/
    petitsingly.

13  Berthold Koletzko et al., "Fatty Acid Composition of Mature
    Human Milk in Germany," *American Journal of Clinical
    Nutrition* 47 (1988): 954–59.

14  J. E. Chappell et al., "Trans Fatty Acids in Human Milk Lipids:
    Influence of Maternal Diet and Weight Loss," *American Journal
    of Clinical Nutrition* 42 (July 1985): 49–56.

15  I. B. Helland et al., "Maternal Supplementation with Very-Long-
    Chain n-3 Fatty Acids During Pregnancy and Lactation Aug-
    ments Children's IQ at 4 Years of Age," *Pediatrics* 111, no. 1
    (January 2003): e39–e44.

16  S. M. Innis, "Human Milk: Maternal Dietary Lipids and Infant
    Development," *Proceedings of the Nutrition Society* 66 (2007):
    399.

17  S. M. Innis, "Polyunsaturated Fatty Acids in Human Milk: An
    Essential Role in Infant Development," *Advances in Experimen-
    tal Medicine and Biology* 554 (2004): 27–43.

18  A. S. Olafsdottir et al., "Polyunsaturated Fatty Acids in the Diet
    and Breast Milk of Lactating Icelandic Women with Traditional
    Fish and Cod Liver Oil Consumption," *Annals of Nutrition and
    Metabolism* 50, no. 3 (2006): 270–76.

19   Innis, "Human Milk," 399.
20   E. E. Birch et al., "A Randomized Controlled Trial of Early
      Dietary Supply of Long-chain Polyunsaturated Fatty Acids and
      Mental Development in Term Infants," *Developmental Medicine
      and Child Neurology* (Cambridge University Press) 42 (2000):
      174–81.
21   I analyzed DHA levels in my breast milk by using a test pur-
      chased from Nutrasource Diagnostics (www.NutraSource.ca).
22   W. D. Lassek and S. J. C. Gaulin, "Waist-Hip Ratio and Cogni-
      tive Ability: Is Gluteofemoral Fat a Privileged Store of Neurode-
      velopmental Resources?" *Evolution and Human Behavior* 29
      (2008): 32.
23   Geetha Cherian and Jeong Sim, "Changes in Breast Milk Fatty
      Acids and Plasma Lipids of Nursing Mothers Following Con-
      sumption of n-3 Polyunsaturated Fatty Acid Enriched Eggs,"
      *Nutrition* 12, no. 1 (1996): 10.
24   Innis, "Human Milk," 398.
25   S. M. Innis, "Dietary (n-3) Fatty Acids and Brain Development,"
      *Journal of Nutrition* 137 (2007): 855–59.
26   B. C. Davis and P. M. Kris-Etherton, "Achieving Optimal
      Essential Fatty Acid Status in Vegetarians: Current Knowledge
      and Practical Implications," *American Journal of Clinical
      Nutrition* 78, no. 3 (2003): 640S–646S.
27   Innis, "Human Milk," 399.
28   Ibid., 399–400. See also Davis and Kris-Etherton, "Achieving
      Optimal Essential Fatty Acid Status in Vegetarians," 640S–
      646S.
29   Innis, "Human Milk," 399–400.
30   Bentley, "Feeding Baby," 65.
31   Several facts in this history of infant formula come from the
      1965 edition of the *Abt-Garrison History of Pediatrics*, ed. Isaac
      A. Abt and Arthur F. Abt (Philadelphia: Saunders), 222–59.
32   Baumslag and Michels, *Milk, Money, and Madness*, 69–70.
33   Bentley, "Feeding Baby," 68.
34   Ibid., 86.
35   Betsy Lozoff et al., "Poorer Developmental Outcome At 10 Years
      with 12 mg/L Iron-Fortified Formula in Infancy." Presented
      orally at the Pediatric Academic Societies Meeting, 2008.
36   *DHASCO and ARASCO Oils as Sources of Long-Chain Polyun-
      saturated Fatty Acids in Infant Formula: A Safety Assessment.*

Technical Report Series No. 22, Food Standards Australia New Zealand, June 2003, 6.

37  Ibid., 3.

38  "Replacing Mother—Imitating Breast Milk in the Laboratory," January 2008, the Cornucopia Institute, www.Cornucopia.org.

39  Baumslag and Michels. *Milk, Money, and Madness*, vvx.

40  Ibid., xxix.

41  Mohrbacher and Kendall-Tacket, *Breastfeeding*, 3.

42  For example, see http://MilkShare.BirthingforLife.com.

43  Jatinder Bhatia, Frank Greer, and the Committee on Nutrition, "Use of Soy Protein-Based Formulas in Infant Feeding," *Pediatrics* 121, no. 5 (2008): 1062–68.

44  www.DustanBaby.com.

45  Buckley, *Gentle Birth*, 136.


## CHAPTER 5: FIRST FOODS

1  Clara Davis published in medical journals, but I haven't seen the originals. I'm relying on several secondary sources. One is *The Family Book of Child Care* by psychiatrist Niles Newton (New York: Harper & Row, 1957), which is mostly out of print but still reliable on family life. The pediatrician Benjamin Scheindlin wrote a piece on Clara Davis, "Take One More Bite for Me," based on her published papers for the Winter 2005 *Gastronomica*. Adelle Davis wrote about Davis in *Let's Have Healthy Children* (first published in 1951).

2  I. A. Abt and A. F. Abt, eds., *The Abt-Garrison History of Pediatrics* (Philadelphia: Saunders, 1965), 222–59.

3  S. J. Fomon, "Assessment of Growth of Formula-Fed Infants: Evolutionary Considerations," *Pediatrics* 113, no. 2 (2004): 389–93.

4  N. Krebs, "Research in Progress. Beef as a First Weaning Food," *Food and Nutrition News* 70, no. 2 (1998): 5.

5  L. Hallberg et al., "The Role of Meat to Improve the Critical Iron Balance During Weaning," *Pediatrics* 111, no. 4 (2003): 864–70.

6  Fomon, "Assessment of Growth of Formula-Fed Infants," 389–93.

7  V. C. Speer et al., "Injectable Iron-Dextran and Several Oral Iron Treatments for the Prevention of Iron-Deficiency Anemia of Baby Pigs," *Journal of Animal Science* 18 (1959): 1409–15.

8  M. AbdulRhman, and N. Tayseer, "Not Giving Honey to Infants:

A Recommendation That Should Be Reevaluated," American Apitherapy Society, June 2005.

9   L. Cordain et al., "Fatty Acid Analysis of Wild Ruminant Tissues: Evolutionary Implications for Reducing Diet-Related Chronic Disease," *European Journal of Clinical Nutrition* 56 (2002): 183 and 189.

10  A. Zutavern et al., "Timing of Solid Food Introduction in Relation to Eczema, Asthma, Allergic Rhinitis, and Food and Inhalant Sensitization at the Age of 16 Years: Results from the Prospective Birth Cohort Study LISA," *Pediatrics* 121, no. 1 (2008): e44–e52.

11  J. Douwes et al., "Farm Exposure *In Utero* May Protect Against Asthma, Hay Fever and Eczema," *European Respiratory Journal* 32, no. 3 (2008): 603–11.

12  Deakin University Press Release, March 20, 2007. Contact Dr. Andrea Sanigorski, Faculty of Health, Medicine, Nursing and Behavioral Sciences, andrea.sanigorski@deakin.edu.au.

13  Lindsay Allen spoke at the 2005 meeting of the American Association for the Advancement of Science.

14  Eric D. Shinwell and Rafael Gorodischer, "Totally Vegetarian Diets and Infant Nutrition," *Pediatrics* 70, no. 4 (1982): 582–86.

15  R. D. Semba, "Vitamin A as 'Anti-Infective Therapy,' 1920–1940," *Journal of Nutrition* 129 (1999): 783–91.

16  Chris Masterjohn, "Vegetarianism and Nutrient Deficiencies," *Wise Traditions in Food, Farming, and the Healing Arts* 9, no. 1 (Spring 2008): 28.

17  K. G. Dewey, "Nutrition, Growth, and Complementary Feeding of the Breastfed Infant," *Pediatric Clinics of North America* 48, no. 1 (February 2001): 87–104. D. Mandel et al., "Fat and Energy Contents of Expressed Human Breast Milk in Prolonged Lactation," *Pediatrics* 116, no. 3 (2005): e432–e435. Published online August 31, 2005.

# Bibliography

Allport, Susan. *A Natural History of Parenting: A Naturalist Looks at Parenting in the Animal World and Ours*. New York: Three Rivers Press, 1997.

*Aunt Belle's Baby Book*. Newark, N.J.: Mennen Company, 1921.

Baumslag, Naomi, and Dia Michels. *Milk, Money, and Madness: The Culture and Politics of Breast-feeding*. Westport, Conn.: Greenwood, 1995.

Behrmann, Barbara L. *The Breastfeeding Café: Mothers Share the Joys, Challenges, and Secrets of Nursing*. Ann Arbor, Mich.: University of Michigan Press, 2008.

Bentley, Amy. "Feeding Baby, Teaching Mother: Gerber and the Evolution of Infant Food and Feeding Practices in the U.S." In *From Betty Crocker to Feminist Food Studies: Critical Perspectives on Women and Food*, edited by Arlene Viski Avakian and Barbara Haber. Amherst, Mass.: University of Massachusetts Press, 2005.

Berger, Gary S., Marc Goldstein, and Mark Fuerst. *The Couple's Guide to Fertility*. New York: Broadway Books, 2001.

Brewer, Gail Sforza, with Tom Brewer. *What Every Pregnant Woman Should Know: The Truth About Diet and Drugs in Pregnancy*. New York: Penguin, 1986.

Buckley, Sarah J. *Gentle Birth, Gentle Mothering*. Brisbane, Australia: One Moon Press, 2005.

Campbell-McBride, Natasha. *Gut and Psychology Syndrome*. Cambridge, England: Medinform, 2004.

Chavarro, Jorge E., Walter C. Willett, and Patrick J. Skerrett. *The Fertility Diet: Groundbreaking Research Reveals Natural Ways to Boost Ovulation and Improve Your Chances of Getting Pregnant*. New York: McGraw-Hill, 2008.

Clapp, James F. *Exercising Through Your Pregnancy.* Omaha, Nebr.: Addicus Books, 2002.

Cohen, Marisa. *Deliver This! Make the Childbirth Choice That's Right for You . . . No Matter What Everyone Else Thinks.* Emeryville, Calif.: Seal Press, 2006.

Cohen, Michel. *The New Basics: A-to-Z Baby and Child Care for the Modern Parent.* New York: HarperCollins, 2005.

Daniel, Kaayla T. *The Whole Soy Story: The Dark Side of America's Favorite Health Food.* Washington, D.C.: New Trends, 2005.

Davis, Adelle. *Let's Have Healthy Children.* Revised and updated ed. New York: Harcourt Brace Jovanovich, 1972.

Eaton, S. Boyd, Marjorie Shostak, and Melvin Konner. *The Paleolithic Prescription: A Program of Diet and Exercise and a Design for Living.* New York: Harper and Row, 1988.

Graham, Judy, and Michel Odent. *The Z Factor: How Zinc Is Vital to Your Health.* Rochester, Vt.: Thorsons, 1986.

Grohman, Joann S. *Born to Love: Instinct and Natural Mothering.* Dixfield, Maine: Coburn Farm Press, 1976.

Groll, Jeremy, and Lorie Groll. *Fertility Foods: Optimize Ovulation and Conception Through Food Choices.* New York: Fireside, 2006.

Hale, Thomas. *Medications and Mother's Milk: A Manual of Lactational Pharmacology.* Amarillo, Tex.: Hale, 2006.

Harper, Barbara. *Gentle Birth Choices.* Rochester, Vt.: Healing Arts Press, 2005.

Harvey, Graham. *We Want Real Food: Why Our Food Is Deficient in Minerals and Nutrients and What We Can Do About It.* London: Constable and Robinson, 2006.

Hilles, Helen Train. *Young Food.* New York: Duell, Sloan and Pearche, 1940.

Johnson, Jessica, and Michel Odent. *We Are All Water Babies.* Berkeley, Calif.: Celestial Arts, 1995.

Kaledin, Elizabeth. *The Morning Sickness Companion.* New York: St. Martin's Press, 2003.

Kittler, Pamela Goyan, and Kathryn P. Sucher. *Cultural Foods: Traditions and Trends.* Belmont, Calif.: Wadsworth/Thomson Learning, 2000.

Kitzinger, Sheila. *The Complete Book of Pregnancy and Childbirth.* London: Dorling Kindersley, 1996.

La Leche League International. *The Womanly Art of Breast-feeding.* New York: Penguin, 1997.

Leboyer, Frédérick. *Loving Hands: The Traditional Art of Baby Massage*. New York: Newmarket Press, 1976.

Lindberg, Marrena. *The Orgasmic Diet: A Revolutionary Plan to Lift Your Libido and Bring You to Orgasm*. New York: Crown, 2007.

Lyon, Erica. *The Big Book of Birth*. New York: Penguin, 2007.

Mittelman Jerome, Beverly Mittelman, and Jean Barilla. *Healthy Teeth for Kids: A Preventive Program: Prebirth Through the Teens*. New York: Kensington, 2001.

Moalem, Sharon, with Jonathan Prince. *Survival of the Sickest: The Surprising Connections Between Disease and Longevity*. New York: HarperCollins, 2007.

Mohrbacher, Nancy, and Kathleen Kendall-Tackett. *Breast-feeding Made Simple: Seven Natural Laws for Nursing Mothers*. Oakland, Calif.: New Harbinger, 2005.

Montagu, Ashley M. F. *Prenatal Influences*. Springfield, Ill.: Charles C. Thomas, 1962.

Odent, Michel. *Birth and Breast-feeding: Rediscovering the Needs of Women During Pregnancy and Childbirth*. East Sussex, England: Clairview Books, 2003.

———. *The Cesarean*. London: Free Association Books, 2004.

———. *The Farmer and the Obstetrician*. London: Free Association Books, 2002.

———. *Primal Health: Understanding the Critical Period Between Conception and the First Birthday*. 2nd ed. East Sussex, England: Clairview Books, 2002.

———. *The Scientification of Love*. London: Free Association Books, 2001.

Perlmutter, David. *Brain Maker: The Power of Gut Microbes to Heal and Protect Your Brain—For Life*. New York: Little, Brown and Company, 2015.

Planck, Nina. *Real Food: What to Eat and Why*. New York: Bloomsbury, 2006.

Pollan, Michael. *In Defense of Food*. New York: Penguin, 2008.

Price, Weston A. *Nutrition and Physical Degeneration: A Comparison of Primitive and Modern Diets and Their Effects*. 6th ed. La Mesa, Calif.: Price-Pottenger Nutrition Foundation, 2000. Originally published 1939.

Reiss, Fern. *The Infertility Diet: Get Pregnant and Prevent Miscarriage*. Newton, Mass.: Peanut Butter and Jelly Press, 2003.

Rose, Amanda, with Annell Adams. *Rebuild from Depression: A Nutrient Guide, Including Depression in Pregnancy and Postpartum.* California Hot Springs: Purple Oak Press, 2008.

Sears, Robert W. *The Vaccine Book: Making the Right Decision for Your Child.* New York: Little, Brown, 2007.

Shannon, Marilyn M. *Fertility, Cycles and Nutrition: Can What You Eat Affect Your Menstrual Cycles and Your Fertility?* Cincinnati, Ohio: Couple to Couple League, 2001.

Singer, Katie. *The Garden of Fertility: A Guide to Charting Your Fertility Signals to Prevent or Achieve Pregnancy—Naturally—and to Gauge Your Reproductive Health.* New York: Penguin, 2004.

Smith, Lendon. *Feed Your Kids Right.* New York: Dell, 1979.

Smith, Lendon H., with Joseph Hattersley. *The Infant Survival Guide: Protecting Your Baby from the Dangers of Crib Death, Vaccines, and Other Environmental Hazards.* Petaluma, Calif.: Smart Publications, 2000.

Steingraber, Sandra. *Having Faith: An Ecologist's Journey to Motherhood.* New York: Berkeley, 2001.

Stoll, Andrew L. *The Omega-3 Connection: The Groundbreaking Antidepression Diet and Brain Program.* New York: Fireside/Simon and Schuster, 2001.

Wechsler, Toni. *Taking Charge of Your Fertility: The Definitive Guide to Natural Birth Control, Pregnancy Achievement, and Reproductive Health.* New York: HarperCollins, 2006.

Wesson, Nicky. *Enhancing Fertility Naturally: Holistic Therapies for a Successful Pregnancy.* Rochester, Vt.: Healing Arts Press, 1999.

Williams, Christopher D. *The Fastest Way to Get Pregnant Naturally: The Latest Information on Conceiving a Baby on Your Timetable.* New York: Hyperion, 2001.

# Index

## A NOTE ON THE AUTHOR

Nina Planck is a farmers' daughter, food writer, and farmers' market entrepreneur. She is the creator of the wildly popular London Farmers' Markets, a gifted speaker, a home cook, and the author of *The Farmers' Market Cookbook*, *Real Food: What to Eat and Why*, and *The Real Food Cookbook*. She lives in New York City and Stockton, New Jersey, with her husband, Rob Kaufelt, proprietor of Murray's Cheese, and their three children. Learn more at NinaPlanck.com, @NinaPlanck, and Facebook.com/NinaPlanck.

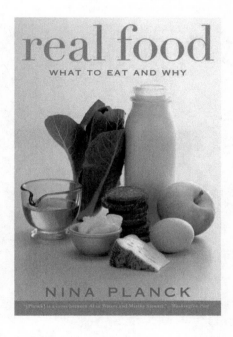

# THE REAL FOOD COOKBOOK

## TRADITIONAL DISHES FOR MODERN COOKS

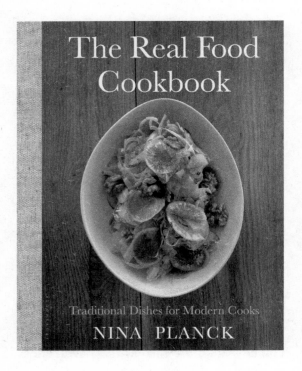

**With over 150 recipes and 100 full-color photographs**

Nina showcases real foods in tempting and straightforward recipes
for the home cook—from drinks and snacks to salads and soups, from
the center of the plate to something sweet. With essays and tips
throughout, sharing Nina's own real-food lifestyle, *The Real Food
Cookbook* provides inspiration for any omnivorous eater.

**www.bloomsbury.com**